MUSICIANS' INJURIES

Musicians' Injuries

a Guide to their
UNDERSTANDING
AND PREVENTION

NICOLA CULF

Illustrations by Harriet Buckley

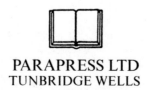

PARAPRESS LTD
TUNBRIDGE WELLS

Also published by Parapress:
Body and *Mind Sculpture* by Josephine Chia
Spanish Dancing by Robert Harrold

Further copies of this book can be ordered from
www.parapress.co.uk

ISBN: 1-898594-62-7

First published in the UK by
PARAPRESS LTD
The Basement
9 Frant Road
Tunbridge Wells
TN2 5SD
office@parapress.co.uk

Reprinted 2004

A catalogue record for this book is available
from the British Library

Printed in Great Britain by
Selwood Printing Ltd, Burgess Hill

Cover by Mousemat Design Ltd. Typeset by Vitaset, Paddock Wood
Print management by Mangrove Production Ltd

Contents

Preface   1

Foreword by Dominique Royle   3

Acknowledgements   4

1. What is an 'Overuse' Injury?   7

2. Causes of Overuse Injury   19

3. Ways of Preventing Overuse Injury   25

    i)   Healthy Practice Habits   27

    ii)   Early Management of Pain   33

    iii)   General Health and Fitness   36

    iv)   Natural Technique   39

4. Which Instrumentalists are Affected?   73

5. Healing a Chronic Overuse Injury   83

Appendix I: Book References/
               Suggested Further Reading   103

Appendix II: Useful Contacts   105

Preface

One of the most terrifying threats to the musician must surely be injury to the hands or arms. In recent years, that threat has become a reality to more and more musicians, and the incidence of playing-related injuries has become alarmingly high. However, there is very little information readily available about such injuries, and most players have only a vague understanding about what they are, what causes them, and how they may be prevented.

This book aims to alter that situation. It was originally conceived as a guide for musicians who are experiencing problems and need facts and practical advice on what to do, but it has become very clear that with so-called 'overuse' injuries, prevention is far easier than cure. It is not only those already in pain, but also the healthy musicians who need to become better informed about the risk factors and how to avoid them. Once an overuse injury is an established condition it is notoriously difficult to heal and can continue for many months or even years, interrupting and sometimes terminating one's playing career. It is therefore vital that every musician, as an essential part of training, learns how to prevent or minimize the chances of injury occurring, to recognize any warning signals, and to control problems if they do arise.

Much of the following advice is concerned with a better understanding and control of muscle tension, and a better understanding of how the hands, arms and body function in their easiest and most efficient way. This has important implications for the musician, because if this awareness can be successfully adapted to the technical demands of one's chosen instrument, then one's technique and music-making skills are also likely to flourish. Stress and tension are probably the biggest factors which stop musicians reaching their true potential, and by freeing the body from unnecessary tensions and developing a more 'natural' technique, not only is there less risk of career-threatening injury, but performance will almost certainly improve as well.

The sources of this understanding are many and varied, and include anatomy and physiology, research into work-related injuries carried out by doctors and therapists, the Feldenkrais and Alexander Techniques, studies in ergonomics, experience with sports injuries, and work by various musical pedagogues who have made natural technique a priority. Therefore this book is by no means a personal viewpoint; it is more a collation of established knowledge from many different disciplines, which can help musicians to make better informed decisions about their work.

The only aspect which *is* personal, is the application of some of the ideas to classical guitar technique, in the third chapter. The modern classical guitar is relatively new as a serious concert instrument, and the technique widely used has led to a staggering number of injuries amongst today's generation of players. I have given some suggestions as to how a more natural technique might be developed and, similarly, it is hoped that readers who play other instruments will be encouraged to think in a fresh way about their own techniques. Although some examples have been related to the guitar, this book is intended for all musicians, whatever instruments they play, and in whichever styles they have chosen.

Musicians are highly gifted people who work extremely hard, having generally chosen to enter their profession through a sheer love of making music. They deserve to enjoy long and satisfying careers, and indeed they could if they learned to look after their bodies with the same intelligence, sensitivity and conscientious-ness with which they approach their music-making. Likewise, music teachers are usually hardworking, dedicated people who care greatly for their students; this book will assist them to care even more effectively by helping them to protect their students' physical well-being in addition to the well-being of their musical development.

Pain and discomfort do not have to be accepted while playing an instrument, and musicians need not suffer the trauma and distress of injury. The ideal for us all to strive towards is a greater understanding and awareness at *all* levels of the profession, right from the very first lessons when habits are being formed, throughout music college and university, and at every stage of the musician's career.

Foreword

As a physiotherapist with a special interest in musicians' injuries, I have worked with many of them over the years and observed the problems they encounter. Interestingly, I have noticed that they are often intensely preoccupied with the sound of the music they are creating, and yet many are quite 'tone-deaf' to the use of their bodies as instruments to create that sound.

Because of this, it is usually only when, as well as the many pressures of being a musician, they experience severe discomfort or problems which have become sufficient to interfere with their playing, that they will venture forward and seek therapy or medical help.

Sadly however, if left too late, symptoms from a playing-related injury can become so severe that they can completely disrupt or interrupt the musician's career, temporarily and at times permanently. This can happen quite suddenly, to the dismay of the player concerned.

A basic understanding of posture, anatomy and physiology (particularly of the musculo-skeletal system), and the subtle interplay of the primary muscles used to create the notes with those that help to stabilise the trunk and limbs, can help musicians to gain a greater responsibility for their own general well-being. It can enable them to find a flexible balance between rest and various activities and so allow them to work comfortably within their own physical capabilities and limitations.

In comparison with the vast field of sports medicine, the speciality of musicians' injuries (or performing arts medicine) is a small but fast-growing one. As yet there is relatively little information, research and advice available for musicians, teachers and health practitioners. A much broader understanding of the injuries incurred and mechanisms involved is essential to all concerned. This book is a thoughtful and welcome stepping-stone towards this, and it serves as both a self-help guide and an information manual.

Dominique Royle MCSP SRP

Acknowledgements

I would like to thank Dominique Royle, who has given me invaluable help and advice at every stage of this study. As a physiotherapist who has taken a special interest in musicians' injuries, she has provided me with much of my source material, has contributed many of the ideas which appear herein, and has spent many hours reading through my early drafts.

I would also like to thank the many doctors, therapists and teachers who have worked with me and helped me in all sorts of ways, each one contributing a unique viewpoint to my knowledge and understanding of this subject.

Sincere thanks to the many musicians with injuries who have shared with me their stories and experiences, and heartfelt best wishes to those who are still suffering.

Finally, I wish to thank all the other people who have helped, advised or supported me; with special thanks to my family, and to Heidi Pedersen, Christopher Clarke, James Eisner, Fiona Harrison, Jonathan Leathwood, Trevor Morris, Amira Fouad, and Richard Williams.

Chapter 1

What is an 'Overuse' Injury?

Numbers in brackets relate to book references given in Appendix I, where the reader can find further or more detailed information.

A<small>N</small> <u>OVERUSE INJURY</u> could be defined as 'damage which occurs as a result of overuse, or inappropriate use, of part of the body'. The hands are particularly vulnerable to overuse injuries, and often become afflicted when a person's occupation involves continual or highly specialised work with them.

Overuse injuries to the hands are especially common amongst musicians, who often spend many hours a day repeating the same specific finger movements over and over again. They frequently have to work from an unnatural and asymmetric posture, and are under a lot of pressure to make their repetitive movements very controlled and precise, even at high speeds. They are pushing the demands on their hands much further than nature ever intended. Playing a musical instrument for several hours a day is basically a very unnatural activity.

In order to perceive the problem fully, it is useful to understand how the hands function.

The skeleton of the human hand, together with its wrist, comprises no less than *27 bones* (see Diagram 1).

The bones are connected to each other at *joints*, most of which allow movement in one direction or more. The joints between the phalanxes of the fingers allow the fingers to be bent (flexed) or straightened out (extended). The knuckle joints (which join the fingers to the hand) allow flexion and extension, and also a limited amount of sideways movement, enabling the fingers to stretch apart. The wrist is actually a network of joints (between the wrist bones, the hand bones and the two bones of the forearm), which allows it to be very mobile and flexible, with the possibility of movement in almost every direction.

In order for movement to take place, a *muscle* connected to the relevant bone must contract or shorten, which pulls the bone towards that muscle, through a movement at the joint. There are altogether *39 muscles* which power the many movements of the hand and wrist; some in the hand itself and many more, both deep and superficial, in the forearm (see Diagram 2 for superficial forearm muscles). Each of those muscles has a specific function, and all the varied movements of the hand require the contraction of different combinations of muscles.

The forearm muscles join on to tough fibrous cords called

tendons, which attach the muscles to the bones. Nine of these tendons pass across the wrist, under a tough ligament which forms what is known as the *carpal tunnel*.

The muscles are activated by *nerves*, which send motor commands from the brain or spinal cord to the muscles, and also relay sensory information from the body back to the brain. The three major nerves of the arm are the *median*, *radial* and *ulnar* nerves. These stem out from the spinal cord at the base of the neck (from an area called the Brachial Plexus), and travel down the arms via the shoulder (see diagram 3). The median nerve passes through the carpal tunnel alongside the tendons.

The arm also contains a complex network of *arteries* and *veins*, which transport blood to and from the area [1].

By observing the size of an average hand and wrist, one can appreciate, then, that there is a lot of activity passing through a rather small area. The complexity of its design means that the hand is able to perform a wide range of movements with a high degree of precision, but it also makes it very vulnerable to stress and strain, especially when pushed to its limits by the demands of a professional musician.

Almost all of the above structures can become damaged if they are over-stressed. The muscles can become fatigued and later damaged; the tendons can become inflamed (tendonitis); the protective sheaths which surround the tendons can become inflamed (tenosynovitis); the nerve or nerve-roots can become compressed by tight muscles or surrounding inflammation; the ligaments between the bones can be torn (sprain); the median nerve passing under the carpal tunnel can be squeezed by inflamed tendons (carpal tunnel syndrome); and one or more of the small bones can be fractured. Several structures may be damaged simultaneously, and there are further complications which can arise as a result of the above. Inflammation of just one nerve-twig or tendon can affect the whole working of the hand, and other tissues can soon become damaged due to the added strain this puts on them [2].

Because of the multiple nature of many injuries, and because the symptoms of the various injuries are often similar, it can be very difficult to diagnose a problem exactly. Therefore, several umbrella-terms have been developed, which can serve as a general

Diagram 1
BONES OF THE HAND AND WRIST

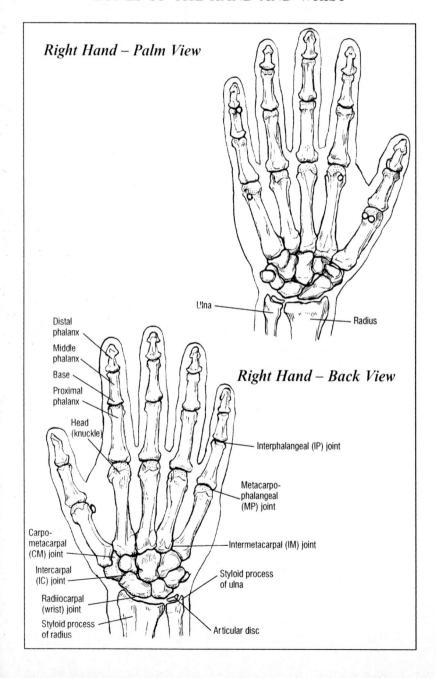

Right Hand – Palm View

Ulna — Radius

Distal phalanx
Middle phalanx
Base
Proximal phalanx
Head (knuckle)

Right Hand – Back View

Interphalangeal (IP) joint

Metacarpo-phalangeal (MP) joint

Carpo-metacarpal (CM) joint
Intercarpal (IC) joint
Radiiocarpal (wrist) joint
Styloid process of radius

Intermetacarpal (IM) joint

Styloid process of ulna

Articular disc

Diagram 2
SUPERFICIAL MUSCLES
OF THE ARM

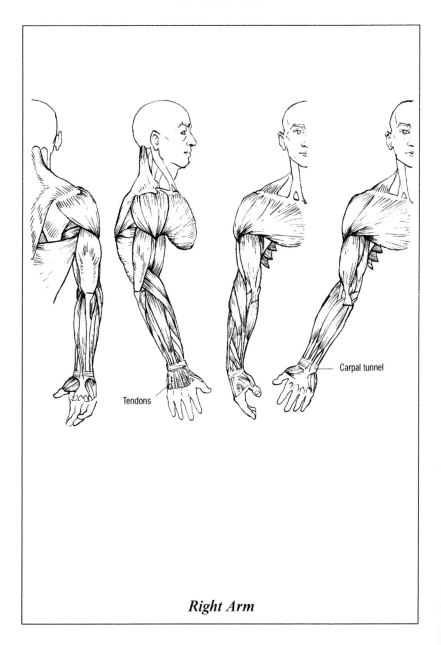

Tendons

Carpal tunnel

Right Arm

description to cover those injuries of the hands and arms (and to a lesser extent shoulders and neck), which are believed to be work-related. These terms include:

Overuse Injury
Overuse Syndrome
RSI (Repetitive Strain Injury)
Repetitive Strain Syndrome
CTD (Cumulative Trauma Disorder)
OCD (Occupational Cervicobrachial Disorder)
WRULD (Work Related Upper Limb Disorder)

Much controversy surrounds the naming of injuries to the upper limbs, and many doctors are sceptical of the newly fashionable term 'RSI' which has been widely adopted in this country. A lot of time and energy has been expended on why this or that title is inappropriate, and there has been no real agreement amongst the medical profession on one 'official' term and a corresponding definition. This has caused many problems with insurance companies, law courts and the like, and has even led some authorities to surmise that 'RSI does not exist'; all of which is very distressing to the many sufferers.

Despite this controversy, it *is* useful to have an umbrella-term which people can instantly recognise, especially since the symptoms of the various injuries can be similar, the causes are often identical, and the manner of preventing them is often the same. For the purposes of this book the term 'overuse injury' will be used.

An overuse injury can be recognised at first by pain or aching in the fingers, wrist or forearm, or by some loss of strength or co-ordination, possibly accompanied by local swelling. The pain is usually confined to one specific location at first. In its early stages it responds well to rest and, provided the cause of injury is taken away and the damage is allowed to heal completely before the hand is used again, the sufferer has a very good chance of total recovery. The problem with musicians and people in other hand-intensive occupations is that they generally do not feel able to stop work, so they continue to use their hands and thus damage vulnerable areas even further.

Diagram 3
NERVES OF THE ARM

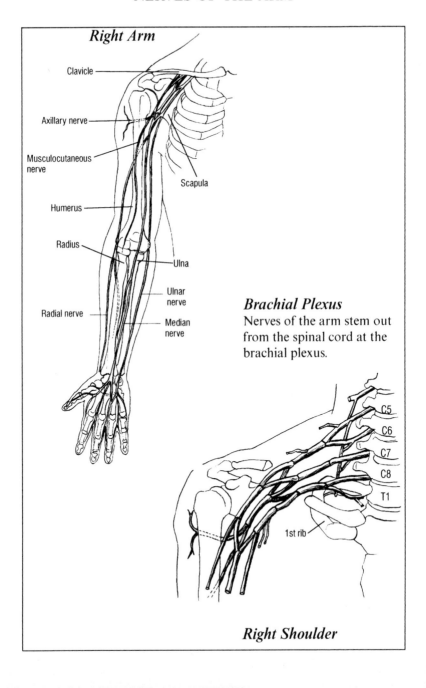

Right Arm

Clavicle

Axillary nerve

Musculocutaneous nerve

Scapula

Humerus

Radius

Ulna

Ulnar nerve

Radial nerve

Median nerve

Brachial Plexus
Nerves of the arm stem out from the spinal cord at the brachial plexus.

C5

C6

C7

C8

T1

1st rib

Right Shoulder

An injury can then develop in many different ways, but generally the symptoms start to appear more regularly and become more intense. Pain may develop in several locations, and the shoulders, upper arm and neck may become affected (though some injuries do remain in one site). Eventually the hand may no longer be able to function, due to debilitating pain and/or complete loss of strength, co-ordination or control. The further an injury is allowed to develop, the more difficult it becomes to treat and resolve, and if it reaches its worst stages it can take months or even years to heal, with some cases never fully recovering.

Every injury is different and it is not possible to predict its course, but a broad guide to the stages of severity an overuse injury may go through is as follows [3]:

Stage 1. Pain or aching is often experienced in the hands, wrist or forearm while playing one's instrument, sometimes accompanied by some loss of strength or control. Pain is usually in one site only, and disappears when the practice-session ends.

Stage 2. Similar symptoms to stage 1, but pain may remain for some time after a practice-session. Some other activities which involve the hands may produce a similar pain. Pain may be experienced in several locations.

Stage 3. Pain at rest, and on many other activities of the hand. Weakness, and impaired functioning at one's instrument.

Stage 4. Continual pain. Complete loss of function of the hand.

In some cases no pain is experienced, but there is a severe loss of control or co-ordination.

An injury may build up over a long period of time, and several years may come to pass before stage 1 symptoms become more serious and start to affect one's work. Alternatively, an injury may develop with alarming speed, and previously healthy musicians can reach a stage 4 injury in the space of 24 hours. All musicians are at risk, throughout their careers. However, there seems to be a particularly high prevalence amongst young female musicians, perhaps because of their smaller hands and limited muscle strength.

The incidence of overuse injuries amongst musicians has become so high in recent years that it is being referred to as an epidemic. In the 1980s, the Australian doctor Hunter Fry interviewed and examined 485 musicians, consisting of four Australian, three American and part of one English orchestra. He found the gross prevalence of overuse injury amongst these musicians to be an astonishingly high 64% [4]. Another large survey was carried out in American symphony orchestras. Data from 2,212 returned questionnaires showed that 76% of players experienced a medical problem that had a serious effect on their performance [5]. There are many more surveys showing similar results.

The really alarming thing is that these high percentages come from surveys which only include working orchestral musicians. It does not take account of the many musicians who have already had to drop out of a performing career due to serious injury.

The increasing incidence amongst musicians could perhaps be attributed to the ever rising standards of performance, which force players to practise more and more in an attempt to become 'better' than their peers. Budding musicians are often encouraged to master impressive virtuosic showpieces at the youngest possible age, at the expense of developing a sensitive, natural technique and good habits of use, which are crucial if injury is to be avoided in the long term. The sophistication of new recording methods has added to the pressure; performers are now born into a world where high quality, technically perfect recordings of great artists are readily available, and musicians often set themselves the impossible task of matching (or even surpassing) these highly edited recordings in their own live performance.

It is not only musicians who are suffering from this epidemic. Other occupational groups include typists, VDU workers, journalists and even chicken-pluckers! At a conference of the National Union of Journalists held in 1991 it was noted that, at the London news station LBC, no less than 95% of their journalists were suffering from 'RSI'.

Clearly, this is a problem which is unlikely to go away unless it is addressed conscientiously and intelligently. In industry, many changes have been made since 1992, when the Health and Safety Executive brought out a whole series of new regulations, requiring that companies take the problem more seriously [6]. Employers are now required, by law, to make an assessment of the risk their workers are under of developing upper-limb injuries. If a risk is identified, then various conditions are imposed which include ensuring the workspace complies with minimum ergonomic standards, and that workers are allowed sufficient rest breaks. In addition, people must be warned of the risk involved, so that they can make a properly informed decision whether or not to take the employment. Failure to comply with these regulations could lead to companies being sued if their workers develop injuries.

Musicians need to adopt a similar responsibility, both for themselves and for their students. The risk of injury is high, the effects are devastating, and there is no guaranteed cure. However, the medical profession is at least in general agreement over many of the causes. Musicians need to learn exactly what those causes are, and try to find ways of continuing their work which avoid as many of them as possible.

Chapter 2

Causes of Overuse Injury

MUSICIANS' INJURIES occur when parts of the body (usually the hands or arms) are overused, or stressed beyond their physiological limit.

Although the word 'overuse' suggests doing something too much, it is not simply the amount of hours spent practising which causes problems. It is usually the combination of frequent use with excess muscular tension or some other form of 'misuse' or inefficient use, which pushes the body past its physical capabilities.

A further factor in the equation is the individual's general fitness and resilience to such stress. A certain set of conditions may not adversely affect one person but may lead to serious injury in another.

RISK OF INJURY =

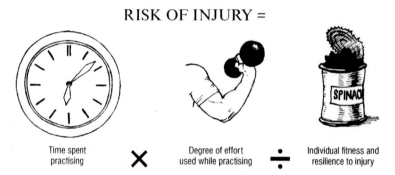

| Time spent practising | **X** | Degree of effort used while practising | **÷** | Individual fitness and resilience to injury |

An analogy may clarify this. If an elastic band is stretched and relaxed, it will return to its original state. If it is stretched and relaxed several times it will probably still return to its original state. However, if it is stretched and relaxed many thousands of times over a long period of time, there is a chance that it will not be strong enough to withstand that stress, and may eventually become damaged and even snap, due to the wear-and-tear of overuse.

Some elastic bands are bigger and stronger than others, so that while one type may snap after three hours of constant stretching, another type may last indefinitely.

If an elastic band is repeatedly stretched with a lot of force, or by something hot, or by something with a sharp edge, it is being 'misused'. That misuse will lead to damage relatively quickly.

Musicians could be compared to elastic bands! Most of the finger movements required to play a musical instrument can be maintained for many hours before injury may (or may not) eventually occur. However, there are certain ways of using the body which can make the wear-and-tear of playing an instrument riskier and lead to injury much sooner [7]. These include:

- Awkward or asymmetric posture
- Sustained or prolonged muscle contraction
- Force (i.e. movements which use a lot of strength)
- Fast repetitive movements
- Raised arms (i.e. holding arms in a continually raised position)
- Deviated wrists (i.e. playing with wrists which deviate from their neutral position)
- Strong gripping action with the thumb
- Playing 'cold' (i.e. not warming up the muscles before practising)
- Insufficient rest breaks
- Undeveloped upper-arm, shoulder and back muscles
- Stress (i.e. psychological or emotional tension)
- Tiredness or ill-health
- Low level of fitness

Playing a musical instrument to a high standard means that several of these widely-recognised risk-factors *cannot be avoided*. Musicians have chosen an occupation which in many ways is uncompromising in the demands it makes on the hands. Bearing this in mind, it is very important that *those stresses which are not absolutely essential, are eliminated or at least minimised.*

Out of the above risk factors come various situations, some quite specific to the musician, which can often cause or contribute to the development of an overuse injury; the most common are listed below. It seems a formidable list, but, as you will realise, all the precipitating factors can actually be avoided.

a) Overpractising

There is a limit to how many hours a day the hands can work without becoming strained. This limit varies from person to person, and is affected by one's physical make-up as well as by one's degree of misuse and/or muscular tension.

b) Poor technique (misuse)

This is not meant in the sense of making frequent mistakes or not being able to play fast; it refers to playing an instrument while the hands or arms are at a 'mechanical disadvantage'. This may be the result of stressful hand or joint positions, unnatural movements, or excess muscular tension. Many first-rate players are not aware of their misuse, and need education in understanding of physiology and body mechanics to realise that their techniques are unnatural.

c) Not warming up before practising

Going straight into fast or demanding pieces puts great strain on the muscles and can easily lead to damage. Athletes and dancers will always perform warm-up exercises before doing anything physically demanding; playing a musical instrument can be an athletic activity for the hands and arms and should be prepared for in a similar way. (That does not mean fast scales! It means slow, gentle exercises which gradually warm up the required muscles.)

d) New use

Muscles and tendons can usually adapt to the work they are required to do but this process takes time. Any new activity should be worked at slowly at first, and time spent on it increased gradually, to allow the muscles and tendons to adapt without risking muscle fatigue and injury. This applies not only to activities which have never been done before, but also to those which have not been done for a while.

e) Doing other strenuous or repetitive activities with the hands

Many musicians develop injuries when they decorate their houses, take up a new sport, or do a lot of writing or typing (to name just three examples). These activities in themselves may not be enough to cause a problem, but when they are done in addition to the workload from playing an instrument, the hands can soon become injured.

f) Change of instrument or technique

Each specialised finger movement is performed by specific muscles. If there is a change of technique or instrument, a new muscle group may be required: one which has so far not been developed. By continuing to do 'x' amount of hours' practice per day with a new technique, a musician may suddenly be working an undeveloped muscle for 'x' hours a day, which could quickly cause strain. When changing instrument or technique, it is important to build up practice-time gradually and provide frequent rest periods.

g) New (more strenuous) piece

If a new piece contains more strenuous chords, awkward stretches and/or difficult fast passages than pieces previously played (or recently played), the hands are suddenly being put under more strain than usual, even if the amount of time spent practising remains the same.

h) Playing under increased stress (whether the stress is related to music or not)

A given workload which causes no problems to a generally relaxed person, may lead to physical injury when that same person is under a lot of stress or is going through an emotional upheaval. Stress causes muscles in the back and neck to become tight and contracted, which can put strain on the spinal joints and emerging nerves. It is generally fatiguing, and lowers the body's resistance to all kinds of illness and injury.

i) Playing with postural tension

This is a very common cause of discomfort, with similar effects to playing under increased stress. In fact, it is often caused by stress in the first place and after a time becomes habitual. Postural tension can lead to a variety of aches and pains, resulting from stiff spinal vertebrae, restricted nerve function, constricted blood vessels, immobile joints and unbalanced muscle tone. The nerves which supply the hand and arm stem out from the spinal cord at the base of the neck, so any postural tension there (as often seen in string-players and pianists while playing) may affect the function of the nerves travelling down the arm to the hand.

j) *Playing through pain*

Pain is a warning signal that the body is unwell or damaged and needs to rest. Musicians who experience pain in the upper limbs often carry on practising, hoping the pain will go away. It will not go away; if something is damaged and is forced to continue working, it will be damaged further and the pain will get worse.

Any one of these causes may not be enough in itself to cause an injury, but when several are combined the risk becomes greater. *The amount of stress on the upper limbs is a cumulative total of all the various factors.*

The importance of rest

One final cause of injury, and maybe the most potent, is pushing the body too far before allowing it to rest. If the body is rested when it begins to tire, it will recharge and after a time become ready to work again. This is one of the miracles of the human body! However, many people in our culture are very bad at recognising when they need to rest, and ignore the warning signals of pain and fatigue, often taking drugs and stimulants like caffeine to mask the symptoms.

Pushing the body past the point of fatigue will usually lead to physical illness, depression or injury. When a musician begins to experience tired hands or arms, a short break from practising will usually be enough to recharge the system so he can carry on again. However, if he does not stop but carries on through his point of fatigue, the tiredness may turn to aching or pain and a much longer break will be required to revive the hands. Carrying on still further will usually lead to injury or damage.

Being aware when it is necessary to take a break is one of the keys to preventing injury. The more risk factors that are present, the sooner the arms will tire and the more breaks will be needed.

The point at which rest is necessary varies greatly from person to person, and may occur sooner when someone is tired, depressed or unwell.

Much of this is mirrored in *Hooke's Law*, one of the laws of physics (see diagram below).

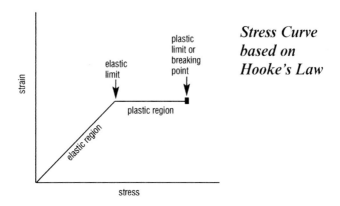

Stress Curve based on Hooke's Law

Hooke's Law states that strain will increase in proportion to the amount of stress. It also states that until the point of *elastic limit*, the strained object will return to its resting-place when the applied stress is taken away [8]. This can be related to the musician in that the hands will tire (or strain) in proportion to the amount of time spent practising and the degree of stress applied when playing. As long as a sufficient rest break is taken before reaching one's 'elastic limit', the hands will return to their starting-place of relaxation and healthy muscles.

Once the point of elastic limit has been reached, the law changes, and the structure under strain will no longer return to its resting-place when the stress is taken away. It is now in the *plastic region*. If a musician continues to practise into the 'plastic region', pain or fatigue will still be experienced when the practice-session has ended. The hands are damaged and will not recover after their usual amount of rest.

The plastic region can lead finally to the *breaking point*. A musician who continues to work when his hands are already damaged, risks reaching his own 'breaking point' when severe, disabling and even irreversible injury will occur.

Chapter 3

Ways of Preventing Overuse Injuries

These can be divided into four main sections:

i) HEALTHY PRACTICE HABITS

ii) EARLY MANAGEMENT OF PAIN

iii) GENERAL HEALTH AND FITNESS

iv) NATURAL TECHNIQUE

i) HEALTHY PRACTICE HABITS

The way in which a musician practises has a big effect on the way his or her body will feel afterwards. Just picking up the instrument and launching into fast scales or the latest piece being learned, and then carrying on playing for long periods of time without stopping, is placing a huge stress on the hands as well as being tiring for the rest of the body. Many injuries could be prevented if musicians developed healthier habits, which should include the following:

Warm-up [9]

Always warm up before practising, as any athlete or dancer would do. Warm-up exercises gradually increase the blood flow to the muscles, joints, ligaments and tendons, which helps to prepare the body for the physically demanding activity of playing an instrument. Properly designed exercises can help to prevent injury and enhance performance:

1. Start with a gentle exercise which uses the whole body. For instance, stand with feet shoulder-width apart, bend knees, then turn torso rhythmically from left to right in turn, letting the arms follow freely.

2. Continue with some broad movements of the arms, away from the instrument. For instance, circle the whole arms backwards and then forwards a few times, bend the arms at the elbows then straighten them out, raise the arms up and down gently, and circle the shoulders.

3. Finally include some movements of the hands, such as making a grip and then fully opening out the hand.

4. After a couple of minutes, move on to some slow, gentle exercises on your instrument, to warm up the muscles specifically required for that activity. For instance, these could comprise some slow scales and arpeggios.

Many players worry that a five-minute warm-up will rob them of five precious minutes of their practice time. In fact, by starting work with supple, warmed-up hands, they will achieve better results, will tire less quickly and will be less susceptible to strain or injury.

Stretch

In order to maintain the natural flexibility of the joints and keep the muscles working healthily, one should regularly perform stretching exercises [10].

While playing a musical instrument many joints of the upper limbs are flexed (or bent inwards), and it is important from a physiological point of view that those joints are regularly extended or stretched out in the opposite direction, which helps to rest the flexed muscles and enables them to work again more readily.

In addition, the body is usually being held in one particular position while playing, often a rather unnatural one. Standing up and doing a few stretches which counteract that position gives the body a chance to release the tension which has built up.

Try to stop after every 20-30 minutes of playing time to perform the following stretches, and always do them at the end of each practice-session or rehearsal:

Hold each of the following *for a few seconds*. Relax for a few seconds in between.

1. Straighten all the fingers (extension of finger joints).
2. Gently bend each finger and thumb backwards in turn (extension of knuckle joints). Use the other hand to hold the stretch in place, but *never go so far that you feel pain*. That advice applies to *all* stretch exercises.
3. Bend wrist gently backwards, using the other hand to hold the stretch in place (extension of wrist joint).
4. Raise both arms to shoulder height, so that your body and arms form a 'T' shape (shoulder joint).
5. Bend the neck forwards as far as it will comfortably go, and then backwards.
6. Turn the head to the right as far as it will comfortably go, and then to the left.
7. Bend the head sideways to the right (so that the ear moves towards the shoulder), and then to the left.

STRETCH EXERCISES

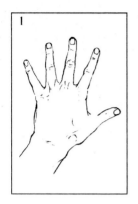
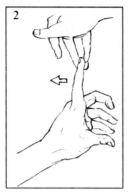
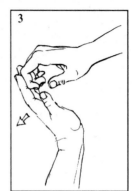

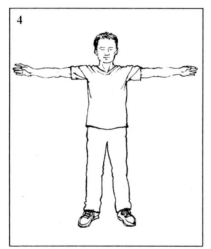

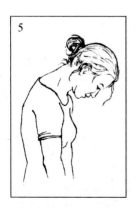
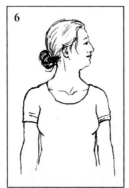
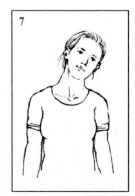

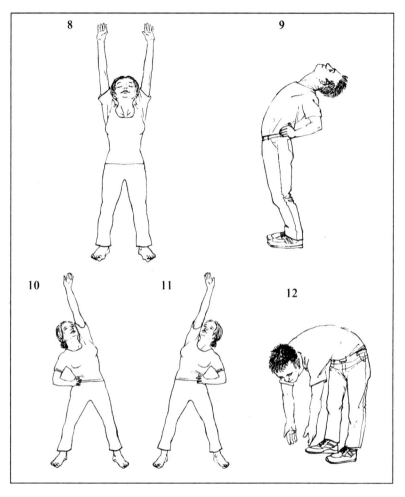

8. Stand up straight, raise both arms up towards the ceiling and stretch upwards.

9. Stand up straight, put your hands on your hips, then arch your back so that you are leaning backwards.

10. Lift your left arm up to the ceiling, and bend your body to the right.

11. Lift your right arm up to the ceiling, and bend your body to the left.

12. Let your body lean forwards and your arms hang down loosely, so that you almost touch your toes.

NB If you already have an injury, then some of these exercises *may* cause or aggravate pain, particularly if nerve damage is involved. If that is the case, stop doing them and ask a physiotherapist for advice on exercises which would be safe for you.

Take regular breaks

Forty-five minutes to an hour is the maximum time one should play before taking a break. Further practising puts an increasing strain on the body and hands.

Rest arms during the breaks

If injury is to be avoided, then the hands and arms ideally need to recover fully before work is resumed. Going straight into another hand-intensive task such as writing, typing, housework or gardening will not allow that recovery. Try to allow some time after a practice-session when the arms can completely relax (this can be achieved more effectively after a few stretches and some gentle massage), and if you continue your day with another activity that stresses the hands, you need to rest from *that* before practising again.

Build up practice time gradually after a holiday or illness

Muscles and tendons adapt to the work they are required to do but, if the activity is ceased for a period of time, they will begin to revert to their previous state. It is therefore important to build up practice time gradually after a holiday, illness or other break from the instrument, so that the muscles and tendons can re-adapt to the task gradually, without risking fatigue and injury.

Do not overpractise for the sake of it

Many musicians feel an almost neurotic compulsion to practise a certain number of hours every day, believing they will lose their ability if they stop for even a day. If they have problems with diffi-cult passages they often repeat them over and over again, in the vain hope that their problems will disappear. In actual fact, they are often practising-in their faulty habits as well as needlessly tiring their hands.

Spend more time working slowly and calmly. If a passage is causing problems, isolate what the cause is, and work out exactly which movement of the hand or arm would correct it. Slowly practise that movement until it feels comfortable and natural, and finally play it up to speed. Shorter periods of intelligent practice can accomplish much more than hours of mindless repetition.

Study scores away from the instrument

If the hands are tired or in pain but you still have energy to work, much can be accomplished by reading scores away from the instrument. In fact, this is a very good way to work even if the hands are not tired. Away from your own technical limitations and the supposed limitations of your instrument, you can hear in your mind's ear how you really want to play a piece.

It is very difficult to be disciplined about practice habits. It is much easier just to pick up the instrument and play. The music and the desire to play can become so powerful that the body is easily forgotten! However, nature has a way of demanding what it needs and, if you try to ignore your body, it is likely to strike back with disease or injury.

ii) EARLY MANAGEMENT OF PAIN

Pain is a warning signal that something is wrong. If you experience it in the hand, wrist or forearm whilst practising, *stop immediately*. Do not start again until it has gone. Gently massaging around the area of pain may help.

If the pain does not go away within half an hour, something has probably become inflamed. Put an ice-pack (or bag of frozen peas) on the area to reduce inflammation, and completely rest the hand until the pain has gone. Put on a splint or sling if necessary, to stop yourself using the damaged limb.

If you get recurrent or persisting pains in the hand or forearm, *seek professional help* as outlined below. The same applies to persistent numbness, weakness or loss of co-ordination. At this stage you may have the chance to reverse the symptoms; if you let them progress any further, you may no longer have that chance. The following points are essential:

- Get advice and treatment from a chartered physiotherapist or other reputable therapist such as an osteopath or Alexander Technique teacher.* Try to find someone who is experienced in treating musicians.

- Ask your doctor to arrange for tests to be done to ensure there is no underlying medical cause such as inflammatory arthritis.

- Re-evaluate your technique with a view to reducing unnecessary tension, particularly in the areas in which you experience pain.

- Modify your practice habits as much as possible and always stop playing at the first sign of pain.

- Avoid or minimize all activities that aggravate the symptoms (these may include carrying bags, turning taps, opening doors, driving, washing-up, brushing hair and writing).

- Avoid pain-killers and cortisone injections; these will only mask the sensation and not remove the cause. It is very important at this stage that you experience your pain so that you know what your limits are.

- Try to relax as much as possible, as stress will aggravate the problem. Massage, gentle exercise and hot baths may all help this.

*See Appendix II for useful addresses.

If the above plan of action does not eradicate the problem, then it is advisable to stop playing completely for some time. This may seem unrealistic to a working musician, but by regularly playing through pain you risk much more serious damage.

If you are a student with recurrent pain, be honest with your teachers about what is happening and ask for your course to be modified so you can take some time off from intense practising. If your teacher does not know how to help you with the problem, seek help from someone who does. If your teacher does not seem to believe you, that is his/her problem not yours! Do not feel pressurised by anyone to carry on working if you have pain in your hands or arms.

If you are a teacher, it is very important to give students a safe space to be honest about any pain they may experience whilst playing. Often students will ignore problems at first, either ignorant of their consequences or frightened of admitting to them.

If a student complains of pain which has developed within the previous week, it is usually possible to pinpoint what has brought it on, e.g. a new tension-habit in the technique, a strenuous activity away from the instrument, or a more demanding piece. By eliminating that element and cutting down on practice for a couple of weeks, the problem will often be solved.

If the student admits to recurrent or continual pain, ask her to stop playing and make sure she really is aware of the dangers of carrying on. Often, you as the teacher are the only person who can arrange for a student to take some time off, by postponing exams and performances, and taking the pressure off weekly lessons. When the pain has completely gone (which may only be after a few days but may take much longer), the student can resume practising, but should do so very gradually and always within the pain threshold. Help her to reduce tension in her technique and make sure she really understands all the possible causes of injury. Above all, do not put her under any pressure to return to full playing too soon. Muscle and tendon injuries generally take a long time to heal and are very vulnerable to re-injury.

A common origin of injury is when a musician hurts a hand or arm doing something completely separate from music, such as sport or home maintenance. This kind of injury also needs rest to recover from just as a playing-related injury would, which may mean suspending practising for a few days. If a player continues with normal practice habits after such a sprain, it never has a chance to heal and in an alarmingly short time can escalate into a serious problem.

iii) GENERAL HEALTH AND FITNESS

A set of circumstances which in some musicians will cause no more than slight fatigue, will in others cause serious injury. One's 'immunity' to various stress factors is largely dependent on one's general health and fitness, as well as the state of one's muscular system. Therefore:

Relax your body and mind

Set aside some time every day to relax your body and mind *completely*. Stress and tension can cause all manner of ill health and are generally tiring to the body. Good ways of relaxing both mind and body include the disciplines of yoga, t'ai chi and meditation.

It is particularly important in preventing injuries that the back and neck do not get over-tense or stiff; massage can be very helpful in relaxing this area.

A useful and easy practice is to lie flat on the floor for a short time (preferably 15-20 minutes), with the head raised on a book or cushion and the knees raised. This is a very good way of allowing the back muscles to relax and the spinal vertebrae to return to their most comfortable position.

Maintain a good posture

Try to maintain a good posture, both at your instrument and away from it. Faulty posture is tiring and can lead to a wide variety of problems. It is a potent risk to musicians, who often have to sit for several hours a day in the same position. In good posture, the spine will not be unduly curved or twisted and the head will be balanced on the neck. Good posture is achieved when the body has a stable base and is in balance, so that no more muscular effort than necessary is required to keep it in that position. The Alexander Technique and Feldenkrais Technique are both good ways of learning about, becoming more aware of, and improving one's posture.

Develop your muscular system

Most musicians have highly developed muscles in specific parts of the arm, but the rest of the body is often untrained and undeveloped. By strengthening the upper-arm, shoulder, chest and back muscles, these can be made to contribute more to one's technique, thus taking some of the burden away from the hands and reducing the risk of injury. Musicians can learn a lot from athletes, who will generally train their whole muscular systems symmetrically, alongside developing the specific movements required for their chosen sports.

Muscle strength can be improved through regular exercise: muscles which have been developed in this way will be stronger, will work for longer periods of time before becoming fatigued, and will need less time to recover between practice-sessions. A woman tends, on average, to have approximately 60% the strength of a man, so female musicians might be particularly interested in developing their musculature, since they are usually expected to perform the same workload as their male colleagues.

Good all-over exercises include aerobics, swimming, and gymnasium workouts. A fitness instructor or personal trainer in a gym could guide you through an exercise routine to strengthen upper-body muscles, which could be performed regularly at home.

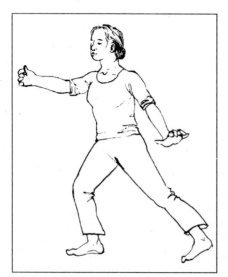

T'ai chi, with its gentle, flowing movements, is a good way of relaxing and calming the mind, while helping to keep joints supple, muscles toned, and internal energy circulating.

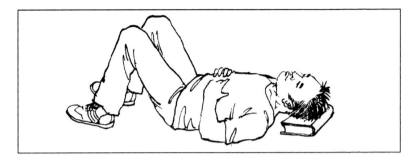

Lying semi-supine for a few minutes is a good way of allowing the back muscles to relax and the spinal vertebrae to return to their most comfortable position.

Eat a healthy and balanced diet

What one eats has a huge effect on one's well-being. When the body is not getting the nourishment it requires, it tires very quickly, and a body working when tired has a lower resistance to illness and injury.

Different nutrients affect different body functions; for general well-being it is therefore important to eat a varied and balanced diet which contains enough of all the vital nutrients.

Keep your body fit and well nourished

Good general fitness is very important to the musician, who often has to work long and irregular hours. She has to find energy and enthusiasm every time she gives a performance, even though many performances take place in the evening, often after a long day of travelling and rehearsing. The fitter and healthier a player is, the more able she will be to withstand stress, and the less likely she is to become injured.

Basically, look after your body or it may let you down. A car-owner will regularly service, fuel and maintain his vehicle; otherwise he knows it may develop problems and eventually could fail its MOT. If your body is neglected, it is likely to develop its own problems and eventually could fail the personal equivalent of an MOT! Unlike a car however, the body cannot be traded in for a new one; it is with you for life.

iv) NATURAL TECHNIQUE

The most crucial factor in preventing injury is a natural, efficient technique which does not put any unnecessary stress on the body.

The following analysis outlines the principles and ideals of natural technique, in such a way that they can be applied to all musicians, regardless of which instruments they play. For the most part, it has then been left to the individual musician to apply these ideals in his own way to the technique of his own instrument.

However, in some cases the general principles have been related to the technique of the classical guitar. These paragraphs have been printed in bold so that non-guitarists have the option of skipping them, although most of the examples and exercises can easily be adapted and applied to other instruments. They provide an example of how one's mind might work when attempting to relate ideas to a specific activity, and may supply a springboard for each musician to think in a fresh way about his own technique.

The basic aim in natural technique is to allow *freedom of expression with the least wastage of physical effort*. The more easy and natural one's physical movements, the less the body will tire and the less vulnerable it will be to injury.

Modern physics sums up natural movement in the 'principle of least action', which states that 'whenever anything [in the natural world] changes, it does so in such a way as to minimize the effort.' [11]

For instance, if a ball is rolled along a smooth path, it will follow the easiest and quickest route, which is a straight line. Similarly, if a brook flowing downstream encounters a large boulder, it will take the path of least resistance and flow around it.

In technique, the musician can follow the example of nature by finding the simplest, most direct and least stressful ways of doing things. Taking away unnecessary tension from the body means that there can be *more* energy for all the other aspects of playing music and that true musical expression can flow without obstruction.

Posture and balance

In creating a natural technique, the first step is to develop a good posture which requires the minimum effort to keep it stable. A good posture is one where:

1. There is a stable base
2. The body is in balance
3. The skeletal structure counteracts the pull of gravity [12].

Gravity is a natural force, which exists whenever matter is present. It gives things weight by pulling them down towards the centre of the earth.

A posture which is *upright* is most likely to counteract the downward pull of gravity and therefore be in balance. A posture which is twisted, leaning to one side or leaning forward will be less balanced; postural muscles of the back and shoulders will need to work hard in order to maintain a stable position.

Posture A

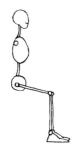

The head is balanced on the spine.
The spine is balanced on the chair.
The body is in a stable position, with no unnecessary muscle tension.

Posture B

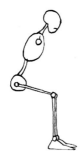

The musician is leaning forward.
The force of gravity is pulling the spine downward; if the player relaxed, his body would fall forward; he must contract muscles in his back to avoid this. The head is not balanced on the spine; the force of gravity is pulling the head forward and down; neck muscles must contract to prevent it slumping forward onto the chest.
Even before playing, a lot of unnecessary muscle tension has been involved.

The diagram showing posture A has of course been simplified; in fact, a spine which is balanced and upright has the following gentle curvature:

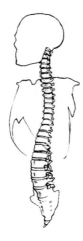

When considering your sitting position, be aware that a regular, flat chair does not provide the best means of support. In order for the spine to be truly balanced over its sitting-bones, and the hip joint to be in its least stressful position, the seat needs to be slightly tilted forward [13]:

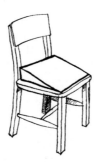

Various chairs have been designed which incorporate this tilt, although at present they are often rather expensive and bulky. An easier and cheaper option can be to place a foam wedge, or a sloped cushion, on to a standard chair, as shown above (sloped cushions can be obtained from 'Back Shops', see Appendix II). Alternatively, a folded towel can be placed at the rear of one's chair, providing a similar effect.

Another factor to consider is the position of one's legs and the contact of the feet with the floor. Ideally both feet should contact the floor in the same way as each other, with as much of the sole of the foot touching the ground as possible. Unbalanced or asymmetric positions of the feet, or crossing one's legs, can result in unnecessary tension in the legs or lower back.

A balanced posture allows the upper body and shoulders to be free, enabling them to support the movements of the arms while playing an instrument. If, on the other hand, the back and shoulder muscles are having to work hard to keep the body stable, then not only will there be unnecessary strain on the body, but the arms and fingers will almost certainly be tense as well.

The ideal standing and sitting postures, then, look something like this:

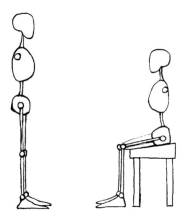

Creating such a posture can be a much more difficult task than one might think, largely because for most people their sensation of being upright and balanced is not very reliable. The spine becomes accustomed to its usual amount of misuse, the surrounding muscles become used to contracting and compensating, and the way a person habitually stands or sits feels so right and normal to that person that he assumes it must be 'correct'. Being shown a better way will often feel very odd and disorientating at first, and in trying to re-create it he will often in fact do something completely different.

For many people, a course of lessons with an Alexander Technique teacher is very helpful in improving the reliability of one's 'sensory perception', and, by creating a more balanced posture on a regular basis during the lessons, it becomes easier, over a period of time, to re-create such use by oneself [14].

Once a suitable sitting or standing position has been established, most instruments have to be either picked up or rested against the body, and the hands must move into position to start playing. Both positions should be maintained in such a way as to minimize stress, since these stresses are going to remain fairly continuous during the playing time.

Whenever possible, the instrument should (like the player's posture) have a stable base, and either be in balance over that base, or be resting against the player in such a way that no effort is required to keep it there. If this is not possible, then try to divide the burden of supporting the instrument evenly between several muscle groups, so that one muscle or joint is not taking the full weight. Avoid holding on too tightly; many players have a subconscious fear of dropping their instruments and consequently use much more effort than is actually necessary to support them.

When playing from a score, position the music stand straight in front and raised almost to eye level. Many players begin with a good posture, but because their music stands are too low or to one side, they gradually twist their bodies or reach out with their necks to get a closer view.

When the arms move into position to start playing, they should maintain the most natural position possible, within the limits of their instrument's technical demands.

In order to experience a 'natural' arm position, let your left arm drop to your side in a relaxed way. Notice that the wrist is straight, the palm of your hand is facing in towards your thigh and your thumb is pointing forwards. This is the most natural and mechanically efficient position, which puts the least stress on the muscles of the hand and forearm [15]. For the purpose of this chapter it will be referred to as the 'neutral position' of the forearm.

Slowly lift the arm up to your instrument, using no more

muscular effort than is necessary and not twisting the forearm in any way. The palm should still be facing inwards and the thumb upwards. Physiologically, this is the optimum position from which to play your instrument. In many cases it is necessary to make some adjustment, but try to make that adjustment as small as possible. The *closer* you can stay to this position while playing, and the *more often you return* to it during a practice-session, the least stress you will be putting on your muscles.

✳

In classical guitar technique, the balance of the sitting position is often upset by the raising of the left leg on the footstool, as well as the tendency to twist the pelvis to the left. This imbalance can often be relieved by swopping the traditional footstool for a knee cushion, or one of the commercially available devices such as the 'apoyo' which can be attached to the guitar to lift it to the required height. Avoiding the habit of constantly watching the fingerboard can also help in avoiding the gradual twist to the left which often occurs when guitarists are playing.

The right forearm should rest on the guitar in such a way that its *natural weight* helps to stabilise the guitar and keep it in balance. No muscular effort is then necessary to keep the guitar in place.

As well as the guitar being in balance, the forearm should also be in balance as it rests on the guitar. If the arm were to relax completely, *it would remain where it is and the hand would remain in its required position over the strings* (Figure 1 below). No muscular effort is required other than that of flexing the fingers to bring them into direct contact with the strings. This ideal balance-point will be the centre of gravity of the forearm in its playing position.

If the forearm rests on the guitar at a point too near to the elbow, its centre of gravity will be unsupported over the front of the guitar and will cause the arm to fall downwards if relaxed (Figure 2). This must be compensated for by using constant muscular effort to hold the arm in its desired position: an option which is fatiguing and limits the control and freedom of the fingers.

If the forearm rests at a point too near to the hand, the centre of gravity of the forearm will be resting somewhere on top of the guitar. The weight of the arm will not effectively contribute towards the strength of the hand, leaving most of the work to be done by the fingers alone (Figure 3).

Figure 1   Figure 2   Figure 3

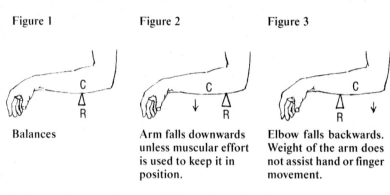

Balances   Arm falls downwards   Elbow falls backwards.
                      unless muscular effort   Weight of the arm does
                      is used to keep it in   not assist hand or finger
                      position.   movement.

C = Centre of gravity of forearm while in playing position.
R = Resting place of forearm on guitar.

On the left side, let your hand drop to your side as already described, then raise the hand to the fingerboard, without twisting the forearm or involving the wrist, i.e. maintain the 'neutral position'.

Because the guitar's fingerboard lies at a different angle from that which the left hand fingers are now in, many players therefore twist or 'supinate' the forearm, bringing the hand square-on to the fingerboard.

Although it has a short-term logic, from a physiological point of view this constant supination is a very stressful position to work from. It is better to stay much closer to the 'neutral' position while playing. It is not always possible to use it, and indeed it is often desirable to move away from it, but it is a very good basic position to return to whenever possible. It is interesting to note that most young children will automatically use it when playing the guitar, unless their natural wisdom is interfered with by teachers! They instinctively know how to use their bodies in the least stressful way.

❄

Muscles

In creating good posture and a good playing position the aim has been to eliminate or minimize muscular tension wherever possible, and to make good use of gravity. Once movement begins to take place, however, it is of course necessary to use the muscles.

Unlike gravity, which is constant and endlessly available, the muscular system is limited because it can tire and is dependent on one's personal energy, fitness-level and build. Some muscles are small and not suitable for a strenuous workload (e.g. the hand muscles), and some muscles, in certain postural conditions, lose much of their potential strength. Before creating a technique, musicians should understand and respect the limitations of their muscles; if not, they may unwittingly overtire them or even damage them, as well as restricting their instrumental performance.

To promote such understanding, a detour will now be made, to explain the function of the muscles in some detail.

Diagram 4 shows a muscle, before contraction and during contraction. Each muscle contains thousands of tiny fibres, which are grouped into bundles. A muscle also contains nerves, through which messages from the brain direct the muscle to contract; it also

Diagram 4

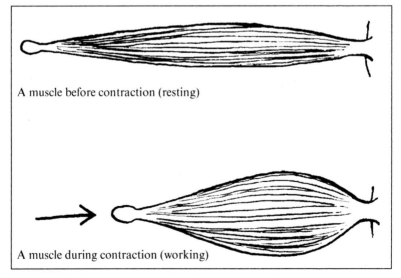

A muscle before contraction (resting)

A muscle during contraction (working)

contains a rich supply of blood vessels through which the blood can deliver nutrients and eliminate waste products. The muscle tapers off at both ends into tendons, which are attached to bones. When a part of the body is required to move, a muscle contracts and shortens, (the result of many or all of its fibres contracting), which causes the bone to which one end is affixed to move towards the bone at the other end.

Once a muscle has shortened, it can only return to its original length (and the body-part return to its original position) by the force of gravity, or by contraction of what is known as the 'antagonist' muscle. In the case of the fingers and arms, the antagonist muscles of the flexors (which cause the joints to bend inwards) are the extensors (which cause the joints to extend or stretch out). Once a finger has been bent or flexed, the flexor muscle can do no more; in order for the finger to return to its original position it is the extensor muscle which must be activated.

This explains why stretching exercises are important between and after practice-sessions; the flexor muscles, which are used frequently whilst playing most instruments, can return more quickly and fully to their relaxed resting state if the extensor muscles are brought into use by fully extending the joints.

A working muscle needs a constant fresh supply of nutrients (including glucose and oxygen), which are transported through the bloodstream. The blood supply becomes several times greater than normal when the muscle is working, in order to fuel the movements and to take away the resulting waste products.

If a muscle is made to work for long periods of time, the blood supply cannot keep up with the demand, and waste products (including carbon dioxide and lactic acid) accumulate. This causes the muscle to ache, as a warning signal that it needs rest.

If a short rest period is allowed, the muscle rapidly recovers, since the waste products can be removed quickly once activity ceases.

However, if rest is not allowed, the muscle will have to work under strain and it will soon become fatigued. The result of this is that it will no longer have as much strength to maintain its contraction, and the rate of relaxation after contraction will be slowed down. If forced contraction is resorted to when a muscle is already fatigued, pain and injury may develop and a longer period of rest will be needed for it to regain its healthy state. Finally, the muscle tissue may become damaged, the tendons attached to it may become inflamed, and symptoms may become chronic. Once the muscles and tendons are actually damaged, the recovery period becomes much longer and the working of the muscle can be seriously impaired.

Muscular action should therefore not be carried on once a muscle is fatigued; a rest should always be taken. The sensation of muscle fatigue is a dull, diffuse ache, felt in the region of the affected muscle rather than in the joint.

There are two types of muscular work:

1. Dynamic effort (a rhythmic alternation of contraction and extension, tension and relaxation, as in walking).
2. Static effort (a prolonged state of contraction of the muscles, as in holding something).

During dynamic effort, the contraction squeezes the blood out of the muscle, and the subsequent relaxation releases a fresh flow of blood into it. The working muscle acts as a pump in the blood system, flushing the muscle with fresh blood and removing waste products. Moderate dynamic effort can be carried out for a long time without fatigue, provided that a suitable rhythm is chosen.

Static effort, on the other hand, is much more strenuous. During static effort, the blood vessels are compressed by the internal pressure of the muscle tissue, so that blood no longer flows through the muscle. A muscle performing heavy static work is receiving no sugar or oxygen from the blood and its waste products are not being eliminated. For this reason, a static muscular effort cannot be continued for very long without strain [16].

The onset of muscular fatigue from static effort will be the more rapid, the greater the force exerted. If the full force of a muscle is used in static effort it will tire within a few seconds, whereas an action requiring only half of the muscle's potential strength can be continued for some minutes. It is generally agreed that, in order to maintain a static effort for several hours a day without fatigue, only 8-10% of the muscle's strength should be used. Of course it is difficult for a musician to be aware of exactly what percentage of a muscle's strength he is using, but, if he aims always to use the minimum strength necessary to carry out a given action, he is more likely to remain within a safe range.

Although dynamic effort is less strenuous than static effort, the onset of fatigue will be sooner if high-speed repetitions are done, or if the force exerted during dynamic effort is strong. Therefore, fast repetitive exercises or fast virtuoso pieces should never be practised for long without a break. The worst scenario possible, is to practise rapid repetitions (as in fast exercises), combined with strong effort (as in big chords or large stretches), combined with static muscular effort (such as postural tension). Such practice is putting a huge strain on the muscles and, if continued for several hours a day, is very likely to damage the hands.

In summary:

a) Musicians must avoid muscular fatigue if their techniques are to be reliable and consistent.

b) To this end, they must:
    i) avoid static (postural) muscular use unless it is essential.
    ii) avoid using more of a muscle's strength than is necessary for a given action.
    iii) avoid rapid repetitions over long periods.
    iv) make sure that muscles regularly return to their relaxed or resting position.

These points will all be directly related to technique during the course of this chapter.

Body awareness

In order that the muscles can be used efficiently in one's technique, it is necessary first to develop a fine degree of body awareness.

The 'kinesthetic' sense refers to an awareness of the muscles of the body, and a sensitivity to the degree of tension they contain at any time. If one is to use just the right amounts of muscle tension to achieve a given result, and to release that tension when it is no longer required, then one needs a very good kinesthetic sense. The following exercises can be used to develop this:

1. Lie on the floor on your back, with your head raised on a book and your arms by your sides. Take a few minutes to relax your body completely. (Deep breathing, warm surroundings and relaxing music may help.)

2. Tense the muscles of one foot *without actually moving the foot*, then relax them. Be aware of whether you are involving any other muscles as well and, if so, try to release them. The rest of the body should remain completely relaxed. (It may take some time to master this exercise if you are not used to such work.)

   Do the same with the other foot, a few times. Always leave some time to relax completely in between.

   Tense the muscles of one foot, relax, tense those of the other foot, relax.

3. Tense the muscles of the right calf, then relax. Again, try not to involve any other part of the body (it is tempting to involve the foot). Continue with the left calf.

   The rest of the body can be worked on in the same way, systematically. Include the thighs, buttocks, back, shoulders, neck, jaw, eyes, forehead, upper arms, forearms, hands and each finger in turn. It will probably take several sessions before you have reliable control of the various muscle groups.

   Being aware of the muscles in the body and of the different sensations of contracting and relaxing them means that you will be much better at recognising when you are using unnecessary tension in your posture, as well as in your technique and in your everyday life. It will also become easier to release those tensions.

4. Still lying down, gently lift one finger of one hand, then relax it again. Repeat the movement, trying to do so with less effort. Be aware of whether any other part of the body becomes unnecessarily involved (for instance the neck muscles) and try to avoid those excess movements. Focus all your attention on how it actually feels to move that finger in an effortless way. How does it differ from the sensations in exercise 3?

5. Repeat with the other fingers, on either hand. Notice the difference in sensation between the fingers. Be aware of exactly where the muscle-contraction takes place (in this case it is in the forearm).

6. Over several sessions, explore all the movements connected with your instrument; remain lying down in a relaxed state. Always work slowly and gently, with the aim being to minimize effort and maximize awareness. It is useful and interesting to work on the whole body in this way, since it is not only music-making which has the potential to improve during the process.

These exercises teach the body how to perform movements with the least effort. It is important initially to re-learn movements *away* from the instrument, because most musicians will automatically react with tension patterns which have become firmly ingrained over the years, as soon as they pick up their instruments.

7. Sit up, and become aware of all the muscles which have to contract to keep you there. Is it possible to release any of them? Can you reduce the strength of contraction of some of them? Are you really balanced on your sitting-bones?

8. Raise the left arm into the position required to play your instrument. Do you habitually contract muscles in the hand, back, shoulders or neck to do so? Most instruments only require a movement of the upper arm followed by a movement of the forearm, in order to bring the hand into playing position.

   Repeat the movement until only those muscles which really are necessary, are being used.

   Repeat with the right arm.

Habitual static tension

Once the musician starts actually to play his instrument, he may unknowingly display static (or postural) tension, which has become a fixed part of his technique and feels completely 'normal'. It can be very enlightening to play in front of a full-sized mirror, or better still make a video-recording of a performance, to high-light one's own habits.

Each instrument has its own pitfalls; it is useful to watch other players and notice those vulnerable areas in order to improve one's own use.

The most common habits of static tension, most of which can apply to all musicians regardless of which instruments they play, include the following:

- One or both shoulders raised or hunched.
- Neck muscles tightened.
- Fixation of eyes (usually accompanied by contraction of neck muscles).
- Facial grimacing.
- Tension in the legs (from unbalanced sitting position).
- Tension in the pelvis (from unbalanced or twisted sitting position).
- Tension in the back (from unbalanced posture or psychological stress).
- Tension in the stomach (often from fear or psychological stress).
- Upper-arm tension (from 'holding' the upper arm in a rigid position).
- Forearm tension and inflexible wrists.

The above tensions should be avoided because, besides their short-term effects on technique and stamina, as a habitual part of one's technique they are probably being repeated for several hours a day, over a long period. The effects of such tensions can accumulate, and even though years may pass without any noticeable problem, the day can suddenly come when enough has become enough and physical pain or injury will occur.

Tension in the hands

Even if unnecessary postural tension has been eliminated, there may still be a lot of tension accumulating in the hands once the musician starts to play. In order to avoid this:

1. The fingers should be independent of each other, so that activating the muscle that gives strength to one finger does not affect the whole hand.
2. All tension used during the production of a note or chord should be released once the note has been played.

The effect of these points is that while one finger is engaged in playing a note, the rest of the hand is relaxed. Different parts of the hand are constantly being allowed to rest and recharge.

Independence of finger movement can be developed through the 'kinesthetic awareness' exercises outlined earlier, and then carried on at the instrument. It should be realised, however, that not all the fingers *are* truly independent, and moving one finger will sometimes activate another [17]. One example is the ring finger, which activates the little finger when it extends, due mainly to the presence of ligamentous bands connecting the tendon of this finger with that of the middle and little finger. Accept these involuntary movements in your technique; they are not actually using any effort, whereas to hold the finger rigidly in place against their will, would do so.

Releasing of finger tension can be developed by practising exercises which use one muscle-action at a time, followed by a conscious relaxation of that action (commonly known as 'play-relax' exercises) [18].

For instance, on the guitar:
  i) Put the left hand into fifth position ready to play one octave of a C major scale starting on the third string.
 ii) Lightly press down the C with the first finger, while keeping the other fingers completely relaxed. ('Play')
iii) Release the first finger and fully relax the muscle which has just been used. ('Relax')
 iv) Lightly press down the D with the third finger, while keeping the other fingers completely relaxed. ('Play')
  v) Release the third finger and fully relax the muscle which has just been used. ('Relax')
 vi) Continue through the rest of the scale in the same way.

vii) When the above becomes natural and easy, the length of the rests between the notes can be gradually reduced, until finally the scale is continuous and the release of tension from one finger takes place while the next finger is playing its note.

❄

Similar play-relax exercises can be devised for all aspects of technique, on all instruments.

Degree of effort used in the fingers and thumb

Carrying on this refinement of muscular use, the next step is to be able to control the exact degree of muscular effort used. The aim should be to *use the minimum muscle energy required to carry out an action*, particularly when considering the use of the fingers and thumbs.

Experiment with reducing effort in your habitual technique, to see if it is possible to produce the same result with less force.

This is particularly important when considering the use of the *thumb*, since any kind of sustained thumb pressure which makes a 'gripping' action is one of the high-risk factors in causing overuse injuries, especially when it is combined with repetitive finger movements. This can apply to playing most stringed instruments, where the left-hand thumb is required to 'rest' behind the instrument's neck but often ends up pressing against it; it also applies to playing many wind and brass instruments, where the thumbs are often resting behind the instrument or helping to support it in some way.

To demonstrate the adverse effect of excess tension in the thumb, carry out the following experiment:

1. Relax the left hand on your lap, palm upwards. Feel the hand and wrist with the right hand.
2. While remaining as relaxed as possible, wriggle the left-hand fingers and notice any change in the wrist.
3. Tense the left-hand thumb and press it against an imaginary

violin (viola/cello/guitar) neck. While holding this tension, again feel the hand and wrist with your right hand. Notice how this movement alters the state of the whole area dramatically.

4. Wriggle the left-hand fingers in this state and notice how much less freedom the fingers have.

In the case of stringed instruments, the thumb usually only needs to be resting lightly behind the instrument neck, not gripping at all. Many players believe they have to press quite hard to counterbalance the force of the fingers, but the amount of pressure actually required to keep the neck stable is surprisingly little, as a few experiments will prove. A good way of developing better control over the thumb pressure is to play slow scales or melodies, rhythmically lifting the thumb away from the instrument neck and placing it lightly back on with each alternate note. Another useful exercise is for another person (or teacher) sometimes to lift the thumb lightly away from the instrument while you are playing, with the aim that only the lightest of touches should be enough to lift the thumb, and that your musical flow should not be affected.

In the case of many wind and brass players, the thumb is helping to support the weight of the instrument, so some tension is going to be needed, but experiment with whether it is possible to use less effort, less 'grip', while still supporting the instrument. It may be possible to attach a strap to it, which can then be supported around the player's neck, making a huge difference to the thumb's workload.

When considering finger technique, it may seem in some cases as though a certain pressure is essential in order to produce a clear note or play loudly enough (for instance), but often the positioning of the arms and hands in relation to the fingers will make a big difference to the amount of effort needed to produce that effect. If the weight of another body-part can support the movements of the fingers, the small finger muscles will not have to use as much strength. Experiment with all the finger movements connected with your technique, to discover firstly whether the same effect could be produced with less force, and secondly whether a slight re-arrangement of position could reduce the fingers' workload.

✳

On the guitar, the effort of the right-hand fingers is largely directed by the dynamic level required. In the left hand however, most players use much more pressure than is actually necessary. An interesting experiment is as follows:

1. Raise the left hand into playing position and place one finger very lightly behind a fret, with no pressure at all. Plucking the string will produce a dull thud.

2. Increase the pressure very gradually until the dull thud is replaced by a buzz. The 'buzz-point' occurs just before the point at which a clean sound is produced.

3. Press just slightly harder and a clean sound will be produced. Is this the usual amount of left-finger pressure you use when playing?

The 'buzz-point', with its unmistakable sound, can be a very useful guide. Practising slow scales and arpeggios at the buzz-point can help to develop a fine degree of control and sensitivity of finger tension. Later, by pressing just slightly harder, the fingers will be working exactly at the point where a clean sound is produced with minimal tension.

Positioning the fingers as close as possible to the right-hand side of the frets makes the buzz-point much lower, so it is important to develop precise positioning of the left hand, right from the early stages of playing.

When playing loudly, it is necessary to press a little harder in the left hand, but not to the extent that most players believe. Experiment with reducing finger pressure at different dynamic levels. Bear in mind that a note played on the guitar has a rapid decay, so although the initial attack may be very loud, within a couple of moments the sound will be much quieter. Therefore, the finger pressure required at the start of a loud note is greater than that needed a moment later; it is possible to release most of the tension almost immediately after the note has sounded.

The minimum pressure required to play a clean note changes at different parts of the fingerboard as well as at different positions and across all six strings. Some players have only one finger action which they crudely use for all situations, thus wasting a lot of muscle energy. *The fingers should develop a sensitivity which allows them constantly to alter their pressure depending on the context.*

✳

The technical suggestions have so far been concerned with muscular tension. The following points concern the *positions* of the hands and arms and the *way* in which they move:

Keep the joints in mid-range

Joints function most efficiently when positioned approximately in the middle of their range of possible movement. From this position, the muscles work more easily and are less vulnerable to strain [19].

For example, the wrist can be bent forwards or backwards to a similar degree, so is at the middle of its range when approximately straight. It is in this position (or bent slightly backwards), that the wrist can function most efficiently. To prove this to yourself, imagine you need to pick up a heavy suitcase; how would you do so? The answer, of course, is with a straight wrist. Try bending the wrist grossly forwards or backwards and then imagine picking up the heavy case: it would be difficult!

The same is true of most joints. By putting any joint through its full range of movement, it is possible to work out what the middle of its range is, and therefore what its most efficient position is.

The further one deviates from a mid-range position, the more stress is put on the joint and the more quickly the muscles will tire. Working from a joint which is at one of the extremes of its range makes it very weak indeed; the joint will truly be working at a mechanical disadvantage.

With joints which are being held fairly static while playing one's instrument, keeping them in their comfortable range will mean that the required posture can be held for longer periods of time before one becomes fatigued.

With joints which are actively working as part of one's technique, it is even more important to use them within their comfortable range, especially when fast repetitive movements are involved.

Once one high-risk element is present (i.e. fast repetitive movements), all the other factors need to be as little stressful as possible
if the risk of injury is to be kept to a minimum.

Mid-range in all the finger joints leads to a gently rounded
hand position, with no sharp angles or straightness.

Be particularly wary of letting the knuckle joint extend (become
flat); this is an 'extreme-of-range' position and as such is very
weak, with the effect even more pronounced if combined at the
same time with flexed finger joints. Mid-range for the knuckles is
gently rounded.

Also be particularly careful when positioning the wrist,
especially when playing an instrument which requires rapid and
finely controlled finger movements. Almost all of the finger
movements are powered by muscles in the forearm which have to
pass through the wrist; if this joint is in a stressful position the
finger muscles will have to work even harder to maintain their
function. As seen earlier, mid-range for the wrist is approximately
straight (or bent slightly backwards), with no prominent
deviations in any direction.

The other joint to be particularly careful about is the neck, one
reason being that the nerves leading to the hands and arms stem
out from its base. The neck should not be stretched forward or
held to one side; mid-range for the neck is when the head is
perfectly balanced on it.

Although the word 'position' is often used, this is not meant
to be regarded as something fixed or static, in the context of
technique. A mid-range 'position' for any joint suggests the place
at which it functions most efficiently, but it should not be held
rigidly in that place. Joints should be flexible and fluid, always
ready to react and respond to the needs of the moment.

Use the stronger, larger muscles to support the weaker ones

Diagram 5 shows the relative dimensions of the muscles of the
body. It shows that, in general, the largest and strongest muscles
are connected to the pelvis, back and chest, and the further away

Diagram 5
SUPERFICIAL MUSCLES OF THE BODY

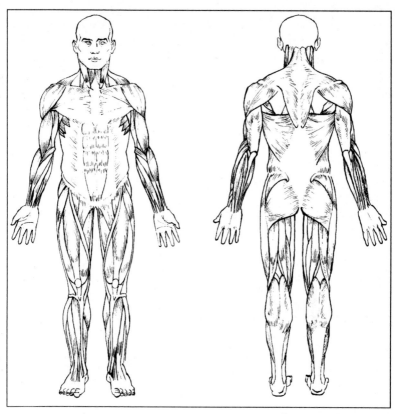

from the centre of the body they are, the smaller and finer the muscles become.

Small muscles have limited strength and endurance and on the whole are suitable for fine precision movements rather than strenuous workloads.

Larger muscles have more strength. An action becomes easier to perform and the movement becomes lighter when the larger muscles do the bulk of the work [20].

While playing an instrument, movements of the *upper arm* are powered by the large, strong muscles of the shoulder, back and chest.

The *elbow joint* is moved by the medium-sized muscles in the upper arms (biceps and triceps).

Movements of the *fingers and wrist* are powered by the small, narrow muscles in the forearm, as well as by some fine muscles in the hands themselves.

It is therefore important to find ways of activating the stronger upper-arm, shoulder and back muscles, in order to assist the weaker muscles of the hand and forearm [21]. A technique which is built entirely around highly developed and efficient finger movements can be impressive in the short term, but it places a huge stress on a part of the body not designed for such a workload, and in the longer term can lead to strain, unreliability and injury. By using the forearm and upper arm whenever possible, a musician can allow the wrist to remain relaxed and fluid, while the fingers are left free to perform the finer precision movements (which can only be done by them), and are therefore much less vulnerable to strain.

There are many ways in which this can be incorporated into the technique of most instruments. Be creative! Most musical results can be achieved by several technical routes; once the focus is taken away from the fingers it is surprising how easy many movements can become and how natural it can feel to play an instrument. Natural movements such as 'jumping,' 'swinging', 'springing', and 'circling' all have a direction and intrinsic strength which usually originates in an impulse from the larger muscles.

✳

A few examples follow, related to guitar technique:

Raise the left arm into guitar position. Hold the arm in a light, poised state; relaxed but not heavy. Nudge your arm, just above the elbow on the inside, with the right forefinger. If the arm is really poised and free, this movement will cause the hand and forearm to move to the right in a very easy way.

In contrast, raise the arm into guitar position and 'move' your hand to the right. Notice how much stiffer the hand and wrist feels with this movement and how much more effort it took.

Go back to the original movement. This was an example of moving your hand from the strong upper-arm muscles. This movement can be used for changing from low to high positions on the guitar. Putting slight weight on the other side of the elbow will move the hand freely back [22].

The above position change could also be made by taking advantage of gravity. Hold your arm in its natural position for first-position playing. Let the upper arm relax (i.e. lose its poise) and gravity will bring it closer to the body, which will in turn bring the hand from the first position to the upper positions if it is relaxed. Open out under the armpit to move the hand effort-lessly back to first position [23].

Next, play an F on the sixth string followed by an A on the first string, without a gap. If this is accomplished by stretching out the little finger, you will be using the small finger muscles. Instead, just move your elbow away from the body a little and move your upper arm upwards, to make the join. The fingers do not have to move at all.

This elbow movement, the 'winging' motion as the eminent violin pedagogue Kato Havas calls it, is a very healthy technique! Not only does it take stress away from the fingers, but it is also a very good tension-reliever for the shoulders, back and neck area if done in a relaxed way. It widens out the back, helps to relax the muscles and lets the ribcage expand so one can breathe easily.

Next, play an F on the sixth string followed by a G sharp on the sixth string, without a gap. To make this movement, play the F from the 'neutral position' of the forearm, then simply bring the elbow inwards, without activating the finger muscles, to reach the G sharp. Compare this relaxed, natural movement with the alternative of tensing and stretching out the little finger.

Much can be learned by observing young children playing music. They will often do all these movements perfectly; they have not yet forgotten how to use their bodies in the easiest and most natural way.

※

Avoid stretching the fingers apart more than necessary

Stretching the fingers apart (abduction) is one of the most tiring movements for the hand. To prove this to yourself, relax the left hand and feel the inner wrist with your right-hand fingers. Wriggle the fingers. Then stretch the fingers apart and notice how tight and tense the tendons in the wrist immediately become. This is especially marked when the finger joints are also flexed (as in most instrumental techniques). From this position, wriggle the fingers again, and notice how much less freedom the fingers have.

On many instruments it is possible to reduce the amount of finger abduction by re-thinking some aspects of technique:

1. Re-finger passages so that the hand is allowed to remain in its natural span whenever possible.

2. 'Jump' from one note to the next rather than stretch out, in situations where this will not affect the musical result.

Of course there will still be numerous occasions when abduction is unavoidable. In these cases:

3. Try consciously to release any build-up of tension after playing passages which contain a lot of stretches.

4. Be aware when you are working on a piece which contains more stretches than usual, and take more frequent breaks when practising such a piece.

The stretches so far considered have been momentary or 'passing' stretches. These should be minimised, but what is far more important is that:

5. The 'home-base' hand position (which is used most of the time) does not include any abduction.

Static or prolonged tension of any sort is undesirable, but when it occurs in the fingers and in particular in their abduction muscles, it leaves the hand very susceptible to fatigue and strain.

Traditional guitar methods which advocate the 'one finger per fret' technique, where the four playing fingers are constantly held over their respective frets, do not take into account the fact that for many players this does in fact mean a constant abduction of the fingers, particularly in the first few positions. Guitarists with smaller hands should not use this technique, and should avoid exercises which demand its use. (It is rare to find actual repertoire which demands it for any great length of time.)

Wherever possible, such players should re-finger passages so that the hand remains in its natural span. For instance, in the first position the little finger can be used to play notes on the third fret. During scale passages, release each finger after playing, and move the whole hand slightly towards the finger which is playing; again this is to retain its natural span.

✳

Some musicians notice that their hands tire quickly when performing a lot of stretches, so they diligently practise 'stretch exercises' in the vain hope of improving their stretching stamina. These exercises usually put a constant strain on the abduction muscles and furthermore push the hands to their limits; a very likely way of *causing* injury! A much better use of time would be to devise ways of *reducing the necessity* of stretching.

Use forearm rotation

In order for the fingers to work efficiently, they should be positioned as an extension and continuation of the forearm muscles and tendons that operate them. If the fingers are placed in line with their respective forearm muscles, there will be a slight change in the position of the wrist and forearm for each finger [24].

This can be seen most clearly by putting a hand in front of you, as if ready to play a piano keyboard. To play a note with the middle finger, the forearm muscles will be aligned with that finger when the hand is centrally balanced.

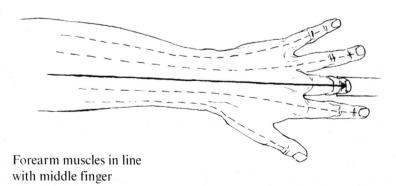

Forearm muscles in line
with middle finger

To play a note with the thumb, there will need to be an adjustment of the wrist and forearm if the thumb is to be aligned with its forearm muscle:

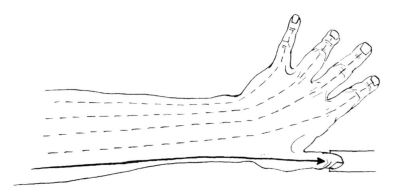

Forearm muscles in line with thumb

To play a note with the little finger, an adjustment in the opposite direction will be needed:

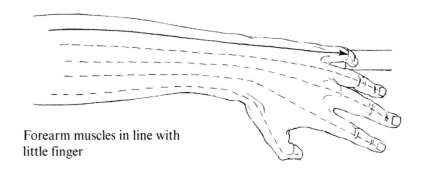

Forearm muscles in line with
little finger

With a flexible hand position, there can be a separate hand and forearm adjustment for each note, so that each finger is working at its position of 'mechanical advantage', where the least strain is being put on its muscles. The balance and centre of gravity of the hand is constantly changing, to support the finger which is playing.

While this is fairly standard practice amongst today's pianists, there are many other instrumentalists who have yet to realise this flexibility. Instead, they develop a rather 'fixed' hand and arm position from which each finger can be used. There can seem to be a short-term logic that accuracy and security of technique might follow from a position which uses the minimum amount of movement, but in fact, because each finger is having to work at a compromise in order to maintain this position, the muscles are tiring more quickly, with the result of less accuracy and control rather than more. This is exaggerated when one's technique also requires the fingers to stretch apart.

The most natural hand positions can usually be formed when one finger is being used at a time; in this situation the hand and forearm position can be perfectly adjusted to support that finger. When more than one finger is used simultaneously, a good practice is to adopt the mid-point between the ideal position for each of those fingers.

Most instruments require a technique which sometimes uses one finger at a time (when the hand can be positioned ideally), sometimes uses more than one finger (when a compromise between those fingers can be made), and sometimes uses several fingers in an awkward or difficult arrangement (in which case just getting the fingers down and producing the right notes must be the priority). A working technique is often a compromise between what would be physiologically most natural, and what the music demands at any time, but as long as there is a balance between the above situations, and comfort of the hands is given priority whenever the music permits, the strain on the finger muscles will be minimised.

On the guitar, if the left arm is placed in the 'neutral position', the first finger is usually in perfect alignment with its forearm muscle. As one moves to the second, third and fourth fingers, there should be a *gradual rotation of the forearm, in order to bring each finger into alignment with its muscle.*

This forearm rotation also serves to bring the ring finger and little finger to their respective frets, without the need for stretching out those fingers. Many players have an unreliable technique which they blame on a 'weak and uncontrolled' little finger; it is not usually the finger which is weak, it is the fact that it is being made to stretch out and play from an uncomfortable angle which makes it unreliable.

Using this forearm rotation, no one finger is being favoured over another in terms of hand position. Each finger has a separate hand and arm adjustment. The centre of gravity of the hand is constantly changing, to support the movements of the fingers. Each finger is working at its mechanical advantage, the need for abduction is minimised, and the larger forearm muscles are being used to support the smaller finger muscles.

In the right hand, because the fingers are much closer together while playing, the forearm rotation needed is much less. In fact, it is so small that in this case a good natural hand position is a compromise between the ideal positions for the three playing fingers, adopting the mid-point. Players commonly make the mistake of positioning their right hands to favour the index and middle fingers only, with the result that the ring finger always has to stretch out. This tension in the ring finger generally leads to a hard tone, an unreliable technique (particularly during fast arpeggios or tremolo), and in some cases injury.

Use of the thumb

For instrumentalists who use the thumb as an active part of their technique, it is important to realise that it has quite a different structure from the fingers. Its base joint is inside the webbing of the hand (near the wrist), and this joint can work in a circular motion, unlike the joints of the fingers, which essentially move in two directions.

If the thumb is used as though it were a finger, i.e. moved from the knuckle and only in a forward or backward direction, it can soon become stiff, unreliable and susceptible to strain. If the thumb is to move freely and keep relaxed, it should move from its base joint, and where appropriate should use a circular motion.

Two further considerations which may be taken into account when analysing technique are the size of one's hands and the size of one's instrument:

Size of hand

Small hands which have to do the same amount of work as large hands are going to tire more quickly and are therefore more vulnerable to injury. Female musicians are at a disadvantage here, with hands which are often much smaller than those of their male colleagues.

Players with smaller hands must acknowledge their limitation and respect it. They must be vigilant about reducing unnecessary tension in their technique, and must reduce the workload of the hand and finger muscles when this is possible without affecting the musical result. The 'traditional' technique may need to be modified and adapted, until it is more compatible with the size of their hands and the stamina of their muscles. Certain areas of repertoire may need to be avoided, for instance pianists with smaller hands may wish to avoid certain Romantic works with their huge stretches combined with fast speeds.

There is no reason why players with small hands cannot become great musicians, as long as they respect their physique and learn how to work around it.

Size and model of instrument

One direct way of reducing the muscular effort required to play music is to use a smaller or lighter instrument if possible. Many instruments have a standard size and nothing can be done to change that. Other instruments, however, have various small adjustments which can be made, which can often make a big difference to the ease of playing. For instance, the effort required to play a piano with stiff keys is much greater than that required to play one with a lighter action. String instruments can often have their actions lowered, making a great difference to the effort required in the left hand. Some woodwind and brass instruments can be made to seem much lighter, by using a strap around the neck to support part of their weight.

One of the golden rules of ergonomics is 'fit the task to the man rather than fitting the man to the task' [25]. Applied to technique, if you are of smaller stature than your colleagues, or if you have smaller hands, use a smaller or lighter instrument!

✳

On the guitar there are several dimensions which are variable:

1. String length: a slightly shorter string length of 64cm or 65cm means that the frets are slightly closer together, so the left-hand stretches are reduced.

2. String spacing: the distance between each string can be reduced, by repositioning the grooves on the nut. This is an easy adjustment to make to any guitar, and can make a big difference to the amount of stretching required in chords and contrapuntal music.

3. Depth of neck: a slimmer neck means that the basic left-hand position is more comfortable to players with smaller hands.

4. Action: the action can be lowered so that the fingers do not have to press so hard in the left hand in order to produce a clean note.

5. Body size: many guitar-makers are returning to the slightly smaller body-size of the 'Torres' guitar. There is no reason why this cannot have the same quality of sound, or ability to project, as larger models.

✳

Relaxation in action

Many suggestions have now been given for reducing muscular effort in one's technique, and for promoting 'relaxation'.

However, once one actually begins to play music, complete relaxation would of course be totally inappropriate! The body needs to be in the right state to be capable of producing drama, emotion, excitement, split-second accuracy and virtuosity. The muscles must be free from unnecessary tension, but they must also be alive and awake, alert and poised; ready to serve the dynamic needs of the music [26].

To demonstrate the difference between the two states:

1. Lift your arms above your head, then slowly let them drop into playing position. They should feel as if they are floating:

freely balanced and supported. The muscles are relaxed, but they are poised and alert.

2. In comparison, let your arms drop to your side, then slowly lift them up to playing position. The muscles are still relaxed, but the arms are more likely to feel heavy, with the 'dead weight' of a relaxed arm rather than the 'live weight' of a poised arm [27].

The posture should also be 'alive'. Although it is relaxed and balanced, that does not mean it has to be weak or static; it can still have direction:

The spine lengthens.
The head is directed up away from the body.
The shoulders widen.
The elbows are directed away from the shoulders.
The wrists are directed away from the elbows.
The fingertips are directed away from the wrists.

All these directions keep the body alert and poised, even when nothing is actually moving.

In performance, there will be times when many of the 'ideals' which have now been outlined have to be abandoned. The hands will be needed in movements which require at times physical strength, at times great dexterity, and at times subtlety and finesse. The basic hand positions will often need to change, sometimes going into grossly awkward shapes. The emotions will probably become involved; affecting the body in unexpected ways.

However: none of this needs to alter the *underlying* state of relaxation and poise, so long as a *well-established, neutral 'home-base' has been developed, to which the player can return whenever the music permits it.*

The definition of 'relaxation' as it applies to physics is 'restoration of equilibrium following a disturbance'. If one's equilibrium is a balanced posture, with hand positions which are mechanically efficient and unstressful to the muscles, and muscular tone which is poised and alert but not tense, then to apply that definition of 'relaxation' to technique whenever possible will help to free the musician's body from unnecessary limitations, and minimize any risk of injury.

SUMMARY

Healthy practice habits

Always warm up before practising, with slow, gentle exercises for a few minutes.

Take regular breaks: 45 minutes to an hour is the maximum time one should play without one.

Regularly stretch (extend) the joints which have been flexed.

Do not overpractise for the sake of it. Practise in an intelligent way; include working with the score away from the instrument.

Early management of pain

If you have pain, stop practising. Do not start again until the pain has gone. Massaging around the area of pain may help.

If the pain does not go away within half an hour, apply an ice-pack to reduce inflammation and completely rest the hand.

If you get recurrent symptoms in the hand/wrist/forearm, seek professional help. Get treatment from a chartered physiotherapist, re-evaluate your technique, and modify your practice habits. If these measures do not clear the problem, it may be necessary to stop playing completely for a time.

General health

Keep your body fit and well nourished.

Set aside some time to relax your body and mind, every day (Yoga, Tai-Chi, meditation).

Try to maintain a good posture, both at your instrument and away from it (Alexander Technique, Feldenkrais Technique).

Develop your muscular system.

Technical suggestions

The basic aim is for a natural technique which allows freedom of expression with the least wastage of physical effort. To this end, wherever possible:

Avoid any kind of bent, twisted or unbalanced posture.

Take advantage of gravity (nature's help).

Avoid extended periods of muscle contraction.

Avoid using more of a muscle's strength than is necessary for a given action.

Use the stronger, larger muscles to support the weaker ones.

Keep the joints in mid-range.

Use forearm rotation.

Avoid stretching the fingers apart more than necessary.

Keep the wrists neutral (not bent or deviated inwards or outwards).

Relax whenever possible, while playing. Good technique has many passing moments of relaxation.

Chapter 4

Which Instrumentalists Are Affected?

I T IS A DISCONCERTING fact that, with many instruments, there are aspects of playing which seem to work against the principles of natural technique. Certain parts of the body's playing-apparatus seem not to fit with the outlined ideals. These are the places which often accumulate tension, and are also places which are more likely to become injured; most structures under strain have their 'breaking point' at the weakest place.

Becoming aware of the location of vulnerable places in one's own physique, is at least one step towards protecting oneself. The first sign of any pain or discomfort in that area should be a warning to stop playing and take a break, and although the workload on that body-part may always be stressful, it may be possible, with some thought, to find ways of using slightly less muscular effort or slightly more natural movements to protect it.

There follows a brief overview of the injuries commonly incurred using different instruments, together with the areas of technique which often lead to those injuries [28]:

In the case of *woodwind instruments,* the vulnerability often concerns the thumb, which often has to support the weight of the instrument. Although it already has a constant role to play, there is a temptation for the thumb to use even more muscular power than is actually necessary to keep the instrument stable, or to 'grip' against it. Problems can eventually arise either in the thumb itself, or in the finger, wrist or forearm muscles, which are having to work much harder as a result of the thumb's tension.

In many cases, it is possible for the thumb to be re-trained to use less muscular effort while playing and, in some cases, it may be possible to spread the burden of the instrument by using a strap around the neck or other supportive device. Bassoonists can attach a spike to the base of the instrument, which then rests on the floor while playing from a seated position; clarinet and oboe 'posts' have been devised; and supports for the flute have been developed.

The stress on the finger muscles becomes greater when the fingers are required to stretch apart as well as make repetitive movements, so the larger the instrument and the smaller the player's hand, the greater the vulnerability. Bassoonists are at risk here, and amongst recorder players the risk is greater with the tenor and treble recorders than with the descant. Size of hand and general muscle fitness might therefore be taken into account when considering whether to play the larger instruments and, if the choice has already been made, players with smaller hands should be especially careful to make the other aspects of technique as stress-free as possible.

Because the woodwind player's arms are held in front of the body, sometimes for long periods of time in the same position, there is a risk of the shoulder and upper-back muscles becoming overworked if there is postural tension or imbalance there.

This problem is worse with the flute, where the instrument is lifted so that the right arm is constantly held in an awkward position, raised quite high and to the right. This can lead to overuse problems in the right shoulder and neck, and/or the finger and fore-arm muscles, which are having to work harder from this unnatural position.

Also vulnerable are the lips and embouchure. The embouchure is working constantly while playing a wind instrument, and often working quite hard and in a way that nature almost certainly did not intend! Any constant and unnatural movement is going to carry the risk of strain. As with all other repetitive movements, the less tension that is used (in this case around the mouth, jaw, facial and neck muscles), the less likely are the problems, and, as with all movements, tiredness or discomfort means that a rest is needed.

Brass instruments involve very similar problems to those of the woodwind for players, although a general tendency to practise for fewer hours per day, combined with the orchestral usage of brass instruments, which usually allows plenty of resting time, means that the stress on the finger muscles tends to be much less.

With a bigger brass instrument, it is usually the act of supporting its heavy weight which causes trouble. General muscular strength and posture while playing are both important things to consider here, and, as with the woodwinds, it may be possible to reduce the problem by using a neck-strap or other attachment.

Perhaps the most restricting problems for brass players are those connected with the lips and embouchure, which are often working very hard and at high pressure. Brass players need to be wary of early symptoms, as these injuries can become very difficult to heal in their more advanced stages.

Singers may feel they are free from the risk of overuse injuries since they do not actually play an instrument. However, the intense and repetitive use of the vocal cords of a trained professional singer is far removed from that which nature must have intended and, as with all intense usage, this can lead to its own problems. Hoarse and sore throats in the first place, progressing to the more serious vocal nodules, polyps and dysphonia, can be the result of intense use of the voice which is combined with postural tension, emotional tension, and/or excess tension in the facial, neck or laryngeal muscles whilst singing.

Violinists and viola players are vulnerable on many counts. Repetitive movements of the left-hand fingers, made more stressful by the raised left arm and often combined with too much thumb tension, can lead to overuse injury of the left hand and wrist, including tendon problems and painful forearm muscles.

Having to support the instrument between the shoulder and chin can lead to overuse of the neck and left shoulder muscles, which can further exacerbate any problems with the hands. The exact positioning of the chin-rest, neck, shoulder, and violin is vital; a tiny adjustment can sometimes make the difference between the instrument being held or being balanced; and the state of the musculature in the player's neck needs to be as free as is possible under these restrictive conditions.

In the bowing arm, overuse of the hand and wrist can also occur, especially if the bow hold is tighter than necessary, and/or the wrist position is too rigid.

Another factor is the constantly raised right arm position. This can lead to tension in the right shoulder which, if allowed to build up, can develop into severe lesions.

In addition, the asymmetric posture required to hold the instrument puts uneven static loading on the spine, which can lead to pain and injury in the cervical region.

It may seem as though these players are doomed to pain and injury! That is certainly not the case, but it is appropriate to be realistic. A player of the violin or viola has many unnatural stresses placed on her body, so it is important to develop the most natural and stress-free technique possible within the set confines, and to be very disciplined about warm-ups, regular rest breaks, general muscular fitness, and the many other safeguards outlined earlier.

Cellists, like players of most stringed instruments, are vulnerable in the left hand to tendonitis and other overuse injuries of the hand, wrist and forearm. In this case it is the combination of repetitive finger movements with a large amount of stretching between the left-hand fingers that can cause problems. The effect is heightened if there is more tension than necessary in the thumb (which only needs to be resting lightly behind the instrument neck), or if more pressure than necessary is habitually used by the fingers.

Overuse injuries can also occur in the bowing arm, as with the violin and viola, although a more natural shoulder and upper arm position means that problems may be less severe.

Playing the cello involves very little movement in the lower part of the body; sitting for long periods of time in this restricted position can often lead to pain in the lumbar (lower) spine, as well as symptoms such as pain or pins and needles being referred into the legs. Sitting on a forward-tilted chair or sloped cushion can help in creating a less stressful position, and players should regularly stand up and move around, during the course of a practice-session or rehearsal.

For players of the *double bass*, most of the problems derive from the extreme size of the instrument. A great deal of strength is required to play it, and the asymmetric playing position makes the stress on the arm and back muscles even greater. General fitness and muscular strength are very important for the double bass player, who is prone to developing back problems. Posture while playing is of course important; many players find it easier to create a better posture if they stand, rather than sit on a high stool or chair.

In addition, both arms may in some cases be affected by overuse injury: the left arm, which requires strength, uses a lot of stretching and is often working from a raised position, and the right arm, which controls the bow.

Guitarists are another group who are vulnerable on many counts. The left arm is prone to tendonitis and other overuse injuries, because of a technique which requires rapid repetitive movements of the fingers, combined with stretching both across the frets and across the strings (sometimes both at the same time), a raised position, and a much greater use of double-stops, chords and contrapuntal textures than the bowed stringed instruments, which tend to involve pressing down one note at a time.

In the right hand, the plucking technique of classical guitarists is often used at extremely fast speeds. This hand is vulnerable both to painful tendonitis, and commonly to 'focal dystonia' in which control and co-ordination of one or more fingers is grossly affected. Although the latter type of injury is usually painless, it is devastating in its effect on performance.

The asymmetric playing posture can lead to muscle overuse in the upper back and shoulders, and the static sitting position can lead to low back problems, especially if the left leg is raised on a footstool rather than using a knee cushion or apoyo.

With all these vulnerabilities, guitarists are another group who need to develop the most natural and stress-free technique possible within their limitations. Balanced posture, efficient and independent use of muscles, minimal use of the left-hand thumb, regular breaks from the sitting position, and healthy practice habits are vital.

For *pianists* and other *keyboard players*, the two sides of the body are used almost equally, and the arms are not unduly raised (providing the chair is the right height), so the task of creating a balanced posture and natural technique is in many ways a more feasible one. However, the way in which the arms are brought forward to the keyboard can cause problems; static tension or rigidity in the shoulders or upper back can lead to pain and muscle overuse in those areas.

Probably the most dangerous factor for keyboard players is the intense use of the fingers. Especially in the case of concert pianists or players aspiring to that level, the finger movements needed are often extremely fast, requiring much stretching, and at times demanding great strength and stamina in combination with speed. Added to this, the high level of competition means that in order to survive as a working pianist it is usually necessary to practise for many hours a day and develop a wide repertoire as well as an infallible technique, often from an early age. The sheer volume of work can put great stress on the hands.

Tendonitis and other overuse injuries can affect the fingers, wrist and forearm on either side (and sometimes both at the same time), commonly causing pain, and often affecting control, strength and/or co-ordination.

For the pianist, freedom in the wrist joint, independent use of tension in the finger muscles, and fluid and supportive use of the upper arms are all important, if the stress on the finger muscles is not to be made greater. Playing from a balanced yet fluid posture, and developing good muscular fitness in the shoulder, chest and back muscles, will further help to protect the fingers. Pianos with stiff keys should be avoided and, for players with small hands or those already affected by overuse, it may be wise to avoid playing a lot of virtuoso and Romantic repertoire with its typical big stretches and rapid finger movements, and perhaps to concentrate more on earlier music.

Percussionists, with their varied range of instruments to move between, combined with orchestral usage which typically allows plenty of rest breaks, may be rather less affected by overuse injuries than some other players.

However, those who practise glockenspiels, xylophones or drums for long periods of time may be affected by the static tension required to hold the drumsticks or hammers, particularly if the player's hold is tighter than it needs to be, or the wrist joints are held too rigidly. In addition, holding the arms in front of the body for long periods of time can lead to painful lesions of the neck and shoulder area.

These latter problems which may affect the orchestral percussionist become more prominent in the case of drummers in rock bands, who are often drumming a repeated beat, almost continuously, for long periods at a time.

Rock musicians in general, as well as players of jazz, folk and other more popular styles, may be affected by similar injuries to those of their classical counterparts. In some cases where players are self-taught, developing an unconventional technique may mean that more stress is being placed on the hands than necessary; a few lessons with someone who is knowledgeable in this field may therefore be useful. Some instruments do not have an established tradition for technique; in these cases musicians would be wise to try and develop their techniques around natural movements and ideals of balance, rather than simply searching for a way which seems to produce the desired musical effect.

❊

Besides the inherent dangers of each instrument, there are also particular risks attached to certain types of work.

For instance, the most intense injuries are often suffered by virtuoso solo performers, who are usually practising for many hours a day, often playing particularly difficult works that push technique to the limit, often travelling and touring with the accompanying problems of fatigue and jet-lag, and all of this while under huge pressure to give an outstanding, virtuoso performance every time.

Orchestral and theatre-pit musicians have their own risks. One problem is that it is not usually possible to take a rest break at the first sign of playing-related pain; the rest breaks are decided by the conductor. In addition, lack of space and seating arrangements may be such that players who are sharing music-stands and also need a good view of the conductor, end up in less than ideal postures. Inefficient lighting and badly designed chairs may compound the problem.

Orchestras often have long rehearsal hours, in many cases followed by an evening performance, and all this happens on top of any individual practising the player may do. This can add up to a large amount of playing, particularly for orchestral violinists, who tend to be in action most of the time during a rehearsal, whereas the other instrumentalists can at least recuperate a little during their rest bars. So much playing can put great stress on the body.

Touring has its own problems: late nights, travelling, irregular meals, possibly less comfortable sleep when away, possibly jet-lag; all making one's resistance to injury lower.

Students at music-college or university are also vulnerable. Many musicians develop injuries at this time, or first start to experience symptoms which may build up and lead to more serious injuries later. For the first time in their lives students are able to focus entirely on music, which generally means greatly increased practice-time each day, often leading to fatigue and overuse. High levels of competition, weekly lessons to prepare for, as well as performances, masterclasses and exams, can put an enormous pressure on the young musician. In addition, this is often quite a stressful time of life, with new and demanding social pressures, and the new responsibility of having to fend for oneself away from home.

Students undertaking academic courses have the extra load on their hands of much written work. Many hours of writing or typing, added to the hours spent practising their instruments, can push these students beyond their limits.

The first few years in the profession can be a difficult time, with the pressure to find work and make a niche for oneself, the high stress of auditions and competitions, and in some cases getting married, having children, and taking on a mortgage, with all the extra responsibilities attached. Many young professionals end up taking all sorts of tiring and badly-paid jobs in order to make ends meet, as well as continuing to practise at home to keep standards high.

At any one time, a musician is in a set of circumstances which affects his likelihood of developing an injury. These include the instrument he plays, the technique he has developed and his general life situation, including his level of health and fitness. These circumstances are constantly changing, so that he is more prone to injury at certain times than others.

By standing back and looking objectively at his own particular situation, the musician has the chance to evaluate what his biggest risk-factors are at any one time. This knowledge can help him to protect himself, to realise when he needs to take extra precautions against injury, and to recognise the warning signals.

All this, hopefully, can be achieved before chronic injury has a chance to take hold.

Chapter 5

Healing a Chronic Overuse Injury

S O FAR, THIS BOOK has outlined many ways in which musicians can help to prevent injury. However, chronic injuries do occur, and for the many people already suffering it is of little consolation to be reminded that prevention would have been easier than cure.

The healing process of an overuse injury can be long, frustrating and unpredictable, often leaving the sufferer feeling incredibly isolated and misunderstood. There are, however, many instances of musicians who have been through injury and, after a period of time, have conquered their problems and returned to playing their instruments, and are now enjoying successful careers again. In addition, it is encouraging to know that there is a rapidly growing awareness amongst both the musical and medical professions about the problems of musicians' injuries and, as time goes by, undoubtedly more specialists will become available, more research will be done, and new ways will be found to help.

This chapter outlines many different aspects of the healing process, and hopefully will enable the musician to understand more clearly what can be done to encourage recovery.

When an injury becomes chronic (stages 3 and 4 as outlined in chapter 1), it is usually impossible for the musician to continue his work. This is a terrifying time, and is rather like a death in that it presents all sorts of practical problems which have to be dealt with, as well as emotional grief, caused by no longer being able to make music.

Despite the turmoil prevailing, it is important for the musician to begin a rehabilitation plan, and to seek appropriate help, as soon as possible.

Ideal rehabilitation plan [29]

Stage 1. A limb which has become severely injured through playing an instrument needs complete rest at first, combined with regular, professional treatment.

Stage 2. Once the continual pain or acute symptoms have subsided, the player needs to rebuild mobility and control by means of carefully graded activities and exercises, in between which plenty of rest is still necessary.

Some normal, 'everyday' use of the hands is healthy during this period, but it is important to avoid any activity which provokes pain or other symptoms.

New ways of using the body usually have to be learned, to prevent problems recurring in the future. These may include a more balanced posture, less muscular tension, and different ways of coping with stress.

Regular treatment and professional guidance are essential throughout.

Stage 3. The final stage is to return to playing the instrument. Because this is the activity which provoked the injury, it is likely to be the most problematic, so playing time should be built up very gradually and always stopped well before the onset of any symptoms.

It may be necessary to modify the technique, using less muscular tension, slightly different hand positions, and a better posture. Guidance from a teacher or colleague who has an understanding of musicians' injuries would be helpful at this time.

Regular treatment is still essential, although different types of therapy may be more useful and effective now.

Treatment

There are many different treatments which may help in recovery from a playing-related injury. These include the following:

PHYSIOTHERAPY
This could include massage, manipulation and other mobilisation techniques which aim to improve the functioning of stiff joints of the spine and limbs. Similar techniques can be used to treat damaged muscles, tendons, ligaments and nervous tissues. Electrical methods such as ultrasound, laser treatment and interferential treatment may be included if appropriate.

Physiotherapy is one of the few therapies which are available on the National Health Service, though limited funding means that sessions in some clinics may be brief and short-term. Consequently it may be more beneficial to pay for private treatment, preferably from a chartered physiotherapist who has specialised experience in treating musicians' injuries.

PHYSIOTHERAPY EXERCISES

A physiotherapist will usually prescribe active self-help exercises which the sufferer can regularly perform by himself. These will vary depending on the precise nature of the injury, but may include:

1. Joint mobility exercises to regain the full range of movement which is often lost through injury, poor posture or abnormal use.

2. Gentle exercises designed to mobilise nervous tissues and help restore normal nerve function.

3. Graded exercises and functional activities to re-build muscle strength.

The exercises can be performed several times a day, and can be very beneficial. It is important to have them regularly checked by a therapist to ensure they are being performed correctly. As a general rule, one should not experience pain as a result of these exercises, though to take them up to the point of pain is often beneficial.

CHIROPRACTIC

This treatment aims largely at correcting deformation or mis-alignment of the spine. Practitioners believe that such deformation may lead to pain or ill-health, often through a resulting disturbance of the nervous system. Radiographs are used in the initial analysis of a problem, and treatment consists largely of a specific form of manipulation which is quick and forceful.

OSTEOPATHY

A similar therapy to chiropractic, aimed at correcting deformations of the skeleton. The main treatment method is manipulation (using a slightly different technique to the chiropractor), but may include other approaches such as muscle re-education and the correction of postural faults.

ACUPUNCTURE

An ancient Chinese therapy, involving the stimulation of so-called 'acupuncture points' with fine needles and sometimes an electrical current, to correct imbalances in the body.

MASSAGE
Treatment which can improve the condition of injured muscles,
as well as alleviating general muscular tension. There are several
different types of massage, including:

1. *Sports Massage*: therapists are trained to treat specific
   injuries, as well as performing all-over massage where
   appropriate.

2. *Swedish Massage*: a neck-and-shoulders, full-back, or full-
   body massage to reduce general tension, usually using
   oils.

3. *Shiatsu*: an oriental therapy, combining Western massage
   and stretching techniques with Eastern massage and a knowledge of acupuncture points and Chinese meridian lines. A
   Shiatsu treats the whole body rather than focussing on a
   specific injury. Unlike with Swedish massage, the patient
   remains clothed.

4. *Thai Massage*: similar to Shiatsu, with some variations in
   technique.

5. *Deep Friction Massage*: this can be applied to specific muscle
   problems such as chronic tension, muscle spasm and atrophy.
   It can be used to break down scar tissue and adhesions which
   may develop following an injury. Deep friction massage can
   be very painful!

SURGERY
With some types of injury, surgery may help or even completely
cure the problem. An orthopaedic surgeon may be consulted, who
will first make as precise a diagnosis as possible, and then decide
whether surgery could be of help.

It is always advisable to have a second or even third opinion
before agreeing to surgery, as an unsuccessful or inappropriate
operation could make the problem worse or even cause permanent
damage. Select a surgeon who is very experienced at treating hand
injuries and in particular musicians' problems, and ensure he
realises that as a musician you will require fine control of all finger
and hand movements.

HOMEOPATHY
This is a system of medicine based on the principle that agents which produce certain signs and symptoms in health may also cure those symptoms in disease and injury, when those agents are considerably diluted. After the initial diagnosis (which may be very involved and include questions about the patient's personality-type as well as a thorough cataloguing of symptoms), treatment usually consists of taking a course of homeopathic pills.

HEALING or SPIRITUAL HEALING
Transference of healing 'energy' through the hands of the giver, often without actually touching the patient. Often (but not always) related to a religious faith, and often given free of charge. Healers are not necessarily medically trained; the healing energy seems to occur naturally in a proportion of the population.

ALEXANDER TECHNIQUE
Lessons which aim to teach an improved 'use of the self', primarily through a better alignment of the head, neck and spine. The student is encouraged to take responsibility for his own health by releasing chronic patterns of misuse, and learning a less stressful, more efficient way of functioning.

FELDENKRAIS TECHNIQUE – AWARENESS THROUGH MOVEMENT
Gentle movements and exercises which develop sensory awareness and aim to improve posture and stressful habits of use.

COUNSELLING
If deep depression follows the loss of music-making, counselling may help the sufferer come to terms with his or her loss.

Different treatments suit different people, and therapists within each type of treatment vary enormously, so it may be a matter of trial and error to find the right person to help. Try to obtain someone who has experience of dealing with musicians' injuries, and who has already had positive results with them. Most people find that it is a combination of various therapies which finally helps them to understand their injuries and discover a route to recovery.

Difficulties

As long-standing sufferers will know, there are several difficulties which can make the above rehabilitation plan very hard to follow.

One difficulty is that most of the above treatments are not available on the National Health Service, and are often alarmingly expensive. This can make having regular treatment very hard for the injured musician, who can no longer play his instrument (or do anything that involves the hands) and has therefore lost his means of income. In industry, workers who develop injuries often receive sick-pay for the period they cannot work, and their treatment is often paid for by their employers. If they are unable to return to work they may be awarded compensation, sometimes of substantial size. Unfortunately, for the self-employed musician these benefits are not available, and this can create a huge problem on top of the injury itself, especially if the situation continues for several months or longer.

Despite everything, try to find money for regular treatment if humanly possible, because without treatment the injury will probably continue for longer, and is less likely to be fully cured. It may be possible to receive financial help from charities such as the Musicians' Benevolent Fund*, and many therapists will work for reduced fees if they realise you are in genuine hardship, particularly if they have an interest in music.

A second difficulty is that of sufficiently resting the injured part, and avoiding tasks which provoke symptoms. If a limb is severely injured, it may be very weak and have very limited function. Almost *any* task may be too strenuous for it, and cause pain. In this situation, a full-time carer would be helpful, to look after the injured musician and allow her to rest her arms! However, for most people that is not an option, and the daily necessities of opening doors, turning on taps, writing, cooking, washing, cleaning, shopping, driving and countless other tasks, can mean that the injury is continually being strained. Every time further pain is provoked the limb is damaged further, and in these circumstances it may never get the chance to rest and recover.

*See Appendix II

Unfortunately there is often no perfect solution to this, but with some careful thought and planning the problem can be minimised:

- If one hand is still healthy, try to devise ways of doing daily chores with that hand alone. Things will usually take twice as long and require some intelligent forethought, but all that is worth it if the injury lessens as a result.

- In the case of the above, be very aware of any developing problems in the 'good' arm. Suddenly, one arm is being used for all tasks where previously they were shared, and it becomes very vulnerable to strain. If any symptoms do develop, make rest a priority; two injured arms are *much* more difficult to manage with than one.

- Ask people for help when it is available. Sufferers are often too proud to ask; however most people enjoy helping others and are happy to do so. Ask people to open doors, carry bags, open tins and bottles, help with cleaning and shopping, etc. Wearing a splint or sling when out of the home makes it easier to ask for help.

- Visit a disabled-living shop or get a mail-order catalogue for people with disabilities (see Appendix II). Here you will find all sorts of gadgets and other aids which can make daily life more manageable for people with limited use of the arms.

- Carry belongings in a bag over the shoulder, a rucksack on the back, or a bag on wheels.

- Eat ready-made meals to avoid having to prepare food.

- Choose meals where very little cutting is necessary.

- Buy small saucepans and light plates, to ease carrying and washing-up.

- Use light or plastic cutlery.

- Drink from a straw to avoid having to pick up heavy cups.

- Bail water into the kettle to avoid picking it up.

- Keep hair very short or in a style which does not need to be blow-dried.

- Use a telephone which does not require the receiver to be picked up.

- Use a book-rest when reading.

The above list is just a start! Be aware of which activities affect your particular injury, and try to devise similar ways of working around them.

The most difficult problem of all can be resting the arms from playing the instrument. Most musicians have been used to playing their instruments for several hours a day, for as long as they can remember. They love playing, and are usually psychologically addicted to it! It is often the one thing they are really good at, and the one time when they feel completely secure and in control. In fact, their whole identity is usually bound up with their existence as musicians, and taking that away will often lead to confusion, depression and a severe identity crisis.

Bearing all that in mind, it can be extremely hard for the musician to put away his instrument and rest for any length of time. The minute things feel a bit better he usually rushes to it and starts playing, hoping everything will have returned to normal. In his enthusiasm and passion, he will rarely start with a couple of simple exercises and then rest; he is much more likely to get carried away and play his favourite concert repertoire, which will almost certainly set back any progress made.

The effects of continuing to play with a badly damaged hand or arm are disastrous. The only solution may be to leave the instrument with a friend at first; preferably a friend who lives too far away to reach without some forward planning and reasonable thought. When the musician is ready to start playing again, it can be useful to use an alarm-clock so that the initial practice-sessions are carefully timed, with no risk of getting carried away in the heat of the moment.

Problems of long-term injuries

Because of the difficulties outlined above, many injuries last much longer than they might under ideal conditions, and can even get worse as they are constantly re-invoked.

Once an injury has continued for several months, further complications can arise as a result of its long duration. These include adhesions (where layers of different body-tissues become bound together due to chronic inflammation or microtrauma), contraction of the capsule surrounding a joint, scar tissue (which may be present in soft tissues as a result of past injury), and atrophy (or wasting) of muscles which are no longer being used.

These problems can become as debilitating as the original injury, and may even remain after the original problem has healed. They need to be professionally treated if normal functioning is to return. This again stresses the need for regular treatment, even when an injury has continued for a long time and does not seem to be lessening.

Returning to the instrument

After an injury, it may be a long time before the symptoms have cleared and the hands are ready to re-train at the instrument. When that time comes, the way in which one returns to playing is crucial.

At first, it is important that the practice-sessions are built up gradually and carefully, with an acute awareness of the body and of any problems which may re-emerge. Start by playing for one minute, and if that does not provoke any symptoms, try another minute later in the day. Progress to two minutes at a time and, in the weeks that follow, slowly build up the length of sessions and the number of sessions each day. Always stop playing at the first sign of any discomfort, with the real aim being to stop before any symptoms arise. Be aware that it is rare for an injury to be healed steadily and predictably; some days one may seem to be moving backwards rather than forwards, so any 'grand plan' will need to be very flexible.

It is very likely that some modifications will need to be made to the playing technique. If the technique previously used was one factor which led to injury, it is likely that returning to it will lead to a recurrence of the problem.

With this in mind, analyse every aspect of technique (not just the specific area of your injury), and aim to modify any action which could be performed with less tension. Experiment with different hand, arm and body positions (preferably under the guidance of a therapist or specialist teacher/colleague), always searching for less stressful movements and more balanced postures. A positive thought is that this is a rare opportunity to discover and develop a truly natural technique, since any unnecessary tension or stressful joint positions will probably cause pain or other symptoms during this vulnerable period.

As well as building up the length of practice-sessions gradually and making adjustments to the technique, it is also important to re-learn the technique methodically, following its natural order of development [30]. This can be frustrating to a musician who has reached an advanced standard of playing and is impatient to return to it; but if the rehabilitation is to be successful and the modified technique is to become natural, then all the movements and techniques required to play the instrument must be re-learned in the same logical order, and with the same care, that a child would learn them. Rushing to regain virtuosity, and missing out on vital stages of development, may overburden the playing-mechanism and lead to a relapse.

A successful return to playing one's instrument requires great patience. It cannot be forced or hurried; pushing too far or too fast will generally have an adverse effect. Progress may be affected by many things, not only work at the instrument. It is very easy to become disheartened along the way and lose one's optimism! However, there are many examples of musicians who have rebuilt their technique after injury, and have successfully resumed their playing careers.

Self-help and the 'Art of Changing' [31]

In order for true healing to occur, the musician must change the faulty conditions which led to injury in the first place.

A good therapist will treat the physical symptoms and may even 'cure' them for a while, but if the musician carries on with the same habits as before, the problem is likely to return.

Each individual must therefore attempt to discover *why* she developed an injury; what were the faulty conditions which led to her problem?

1. What were the contributing factors which may have been present for a long time?

2. What were the precipitating factors which finally tipped the balance?

As a result of this, the musician can make a list of:

3. Factors which need to change if she is to be healed,

4. Factors which need to change if she is to play her instrument again.

The answers to these questions may be purely practical and physical, or they may go deeper and involve the emotions and the psyche. When an injury has reached the stage where it causes inability to function at the instrument, the answers will probably not be simple! There may be several overlapping and possibly deep-rooted problems, all of which have to be acknowledged and worked at. Musicians have often neglected or ignored their bodies for years, and in order to recover they often need muscular re-education, postural re-education, stress management, treatment of various physical problems, and psychological help as well.

One of the biggest problems here, is that most people are not aware of their destructive habits (whether muscular, postural, emotional or psychological). However obvious these may be to other people, they feel completely normal to the person involved! For instance, many musicians who suffer injuries have a generally high level of muscular tension in their whole bodies, as well as an inappropriate amount of tension in the muscles required to play their instruments. However, because they rarely (if ever) experience anything different, they honestly believe they are relaxed.

Healing requires that the injured musician is open to the possibility that the way he is functioning may be limiting his progress; that something he is actually *doing* may be causing the problem. He needs to be open to the idea that there may be a different and better way to learn.

Once the faulty or misguided habits have been recognised (or pointed out by a therapist), it can still be very difficult to change them. The way a person acts is generally firmly ingrained, and the process of changing will usually require the patient help of an

Alexander Technique teacher, counsellor or other therapist, often over a long period of time.

At first, any change may feel 'wrong' and uncomfortable, simply because it is unfamiliar. For instance, if a person is used to tilting his head to the right most of the time, having his head balanced correctly on his neck by a therapist will feel 'wrong' at first; the patient will believe he must now be tilting his head to the left. Soon after leaving the therapist's room he will probably have a strong urge to tilt his head back to the right, in order to feel 'normal' again.

In some cases, changing a habit or releasing a habitual tension may be unsettling, disturbing or even frightening. Many of one's tensions originate in traumatic experiences from childhood or adolescence; releasing the tension may also release those traumas, along with the emotions which have been locked into the body ever since.

There are many different levels on which one can change.

If an injury is not improving, the sufferer may have to ask himself if he has changed *enough* to allow healing to occur. Is it necessary to change on a different level?

The 'art of changing' is a challenging one, requiring courage, wisdom, a spirit of adventure, and a readiness to learn from the obstacles which seem to bar the way ahead. Injury is often a time of deep searching and profound change, which may affect the course of the rest of one's life.

Creative visualisation

In some cases, the mind may be limiting the process of healing, through mental blocks, fears, or rigid patterns of thought. A very useful technique which can help to alter such patterns is 'creative visualisation'. Basically, this is a form of positive thinking, usually done from a very relaxed state when the subconscious mind is most receptive to change.

As an experiment, sit or lie down quietly, and imagine playing the instrument without pain or other symptoms. This may be surprisingly difficult to do after a long injury, and shows that the mind can be very powerful in anticipating pain which has become habitual.

If the above exercise proves impossible, then there is little chance of actually playing the instrument without pain! In this case, try the following three visualisations, which have been devised to alter that pattern of thought in a gradual and reassuring way. Take as long as you like over each exercise, pausing to relax and breathe calmly between each instruction. A particularly good way of doing the exercises is to record the directions in a calm, soothing voice, perhaps with some gentle music in the background, then play the cassette back as you relax:

VISUALISATION 1a
Lie down in a comfortable position and relax for a few minutes ...
When you feel relaxed, try to imagine you are lying on a soft, sandy beach, on a warm summer's afternoon ...
The sea is calm and inviting ...
Gently run your hands through the sand a few times, feeling the grains fall between your fingers ...
Notice that the sensation in each arm is the same; no pain or other symptoms are present ...
Relax.

When this can be done comfortably, try visualising something that would be more physically strenuous for the arms, but still avoiding any connection to music or your instrument:

VISUALISATION 1b
Lie down in a comfortable position and breathe deeply for a couple of minutes ...
When you feel relaxed, try to imagine you are at a farm in the country, on a beautiful summer's day ...
There are vegetables planted nearby, which need fresh water ...
Walk over to an outside tap, and fill up two pails of water from this tap ...
Pick up a full pail with one hand; there is no pain ...
Pick up the second pail with your other hand; there is still no pain ...
Carry the pails over to the vegetables and water them ...
Relax.

If this exercise provokes any symptoms, try to notice what it is (if anything) that you habitually do when you anticipate using the injured arm. It may be that you tense a group of muscles without realising, allowing part of your body to become tight. Once you have become aware of this, try to inhibit your usual response. Aim for a deeper and deeper level of relaxation, until the muscles connected with your injury are calm.

When this has been mastered, build up to visualising playing your instrument:

VISUALISATION 1c
Find a warm, comfortable position, and relax ...
Imagine picking up your instrument and looking at it. You feel relaxed and happy, and admire the beauty of your instrument ...
Sit with your instrument in the playing position, and notice that there is no pain or discomfort in your body ...
Begin to play a slow, quiet scale, in a very relaxed manner. Your hands and arms feel comfortable and natural ...
Move on to playing a piece of music. Playing is an enjoyable experience for the body; no pain or discomfort is present ...
Relax.

If the above exercises proved helpful, there are many other ways in which creative visualisations can be used to assist the healing process. Some musicians are sceptical and suspicious of what they consider to be rather 'new-age' methods, and others do not find it easy to conjure up visual images, but many people with physical problems experience a real change when they use them regularly. The mind can be a very powerful tool, and a positive outlook, combined with a strong belief that healing will take place, can have a profound effect on the body [32].

The following three exercises have been designed to help the sufferer release some of the pain and muscle tension associated with an overuse injury:

VISUALISATION 2
Lie in a comfortable position and relax …
Breathe in deeply, and as you breathe out, purse your lips so that you exhale slowly, making a gentle sound …
With each further exhalation, imagine all the pain and tension in your body is being pushed down through your arms and leaving through the tips of your fingers …
Repeat several times until all the tension has been expelled and your arms feel comfortable and relaxed …
Relax.

VISUALISATION 3
Lie in a comfortable position and relax for a few minutes …
Imagine a soft, blue light entering your head, and travelling through to your neck …
This is a relaxing light, which makes your head and neck feel calm and soothed …
The light moves across your shoulders and, as it enters your arms, it changes colour to purple …
Purple is a soft, healing colour …
The light travels slowly down your arms to your hands, filling your limbs with magical, healing energy …
You relax, as the soothing light heals you …
Relax.

VISUALISATION 4
Lie in a comfortable position and relax for a few minutes …
Compare the sensations in your arms, and notice the difference between them …
Try to re-create the feeling you experienced in the 'bad' arm, in the other arm …
Both arms have the same sensation now …
Try to experience a pain-free, 'normal' sensation in the injured arm, so that the two arms have now swopped roles …
Relax both arms until no pain is present. Both arms now feel the same …
Relax.

Summary and final advice

The process of healing rarely happens by itself: it has to be worked at by doctors, therapists, and most importantly of all, by the sufferer. Patience and perseverance are required in abundance, along with a willingness to change, improve, progress and learn.

A summary of the key points of this chapter follows, together with some final advice on coping with an overuse injury:

- Relax and remain calm, as much as possible. Although this is a devastating experience for any musician, stress will make the symptoms worse.

- Find a way of securing some regular income as soon as possible after injury; it may be some time before you can work again. (It is often possible to claim Income Support or Sickness Benefit).

- Seek regular, professional treatment.

- Get advice from a physiotherapist about exercises you can do by yourself, and have them regularly checked to ensure you are doing them correctly.

- Realise that the place where your symptoms occur may not be the root of your problem, so treatment may need to be aimed elsewhere.

- Avoid any activity which provokes pain or other symptoms.

- If one hand is still healthy, try to devise ways of doing things with that hand alone.

- Avoid playing your instrument until the pain has completely gone. Always stop practising well before any symptoms re-emerge.

- Try to discover why you developed an injury, and plan how to avoid those causes in the future.

- Analyse (and if necessary modify) your postural and muscular use, your instrumental technique, and your reaction to stress. Try to be honest and objective.

- Avoid short-term solutions such as cortisone injections or strong pain-killers. These can mask the pain and enable you to continue using the affected limb, which may cause an aggravation of the injury and jeopardize its changes of recovery.

- Try not to pin all your hopes on a 'miracle-cure'; this puts an unfair pressure on the therapist and may lead to disappointment for yourself.

- Try to get as precise a diagnosis as possible. It is always advisable to get more than one opinion as doctors' comments vary greatly.

- Seek out other people with the same problem; it can be very comforting to discover you are not alone.

- Concentrate on the things you can do rather than the things you cannot do.

- Find another outlet for your frustrated creative energy, such as singing or acting.

- Remember: most people do eventually recover! Good luck!

Appendix I
Book References/Suggested Further Reading

1. Gerard Tortura and Nicholas Anagnostakes, *Principles of Anatomy and Physiology* (6th edition), Harper Collins, New York 1990.

   Raoul Tubiana, 'Functional Anatomy of the Hand' (*Medical Problems of Performing Artists*), September 1988.

2. Brian Corrigan and G.D. Maitland, *Practical Orthopaedic Medicine*, Butterworths, London 1983.

3. Hunter J.H.Fry, 'Overuse Syndrome in Musicians: Prevention and Management' (*The Lancet*), September 1986.

4. Hunter J.H.Fry, 'Incidence of Overuse Injury Syndrome in the Symphony Orchestra' (*Medical Problems of Performing Artists*), I, 1986.

5. Martin Fishbein and Susan Middlestadt, 'Medical Problems among ICSOM Musicians: Overview of a National Survey' (*Medical Problems of Performing Artists*), March 1988.

6. 'Manual Handling Operations Regulations 1992', Health and Safety Executive, 1992.

   'Management of Health and Safety at Work Regulations 1992', Health and Safety Executive, 1992.

7. P .van Welv, 'Design and Disease' (*Applied Ergonomics*), December 1970.

   Stephen Pheasant, *Bodyspace-Anthropometry, Ergonomics and Design*, Taylor and Francis, London 1988.

   'Work Related Upper Limb Disorders – A Guide to Prevention', Health and Safety Executive, 1990.

8. John Daintwith and R.D. Nelson (editors), *Dictionary of Mathematics*, Penguin, London 1989.

9. Dr. Lars Peterson and Dr. Per Renstrom, *Sports Injuries – Their Prevention and Treatment*, Dunitz, 1986.

10. Wendy Chalmers Mill, *Repetitive Strain Injury*, Thorsons, London 1994.

11. Paul Davies and John Gribbin, *The Matter Myth – Towards 21st Century Science*, Viking, 1991.

12. Moshe Feldenkrais, *Awareness Through Movement*, Penguin, London 1980.

13. Andrew Wilson, *The Complete Guide to Good Posture at Work*, Vermillion, London 1996.

14. F.M. Alexander, *The Use of the Self*, Victor Gollancz Ltd, London.

    W. Barlow, *The Alexander Principle*, Victor Gollancz, London 1973.

15. Stephen Pheasant, *Bodyspace-Anthropometry, Ergonomics and Design*, Taylor and Francis, London 1988.

16. Etienne Grandjean, *Fitting the Task to the Man: A Textbook of Occupational Ergonomics* (4th edition), Taylor and Francis, London 1988.

17. Raoul Tubiana, 'Movements of the Fingers' (*Medical Problems of Performing Artists*), December 1988.

18. Lee F. Ryan, *The Natural Classical Guitar*, Prentice-Hall, 1984.

19. Otto Ortmann, *The Physiological Mechanics of Piano Technique*, Da Capo Press, New York 1981.

20. See 12.

21. Gyorgy Sandor, *On Piano Playing*, Collier Macmillan, London 1981.

22. Acknowledgement to Kato Havas for this idea.

23. Acknowledgement to Ricardo Iznaola for this idea.

24. See 21.

25. See 16.

26. Tobias Matthay, *Epitome of the Laws of Pianoforte Technique*, Oxford University Press, 1931.

    Ricardo Iznaola, *On Practising*, IGW, Colorado 1992.

27. Kato Havas, *Stage Fright*, Bosworth, London 1973.

28. See 4 and 5.

29. See 3.

    D. Royle, 'A Physiotherapist's Approach to Musicians' Injuries', *ISSTIP Journal*, November 1992.

30. Moshe Feldenkrais, *Body Awareness as Healing Therapy – The Case of Nora*, Frog Ltd and Somatic Resources, California 1993.

31. Glen Park, *The Art of Changing*, Ashgrove Press, Bath 1989.

32. Matthew Manning, *Guide to Self-Healing*, Thorsons, Wellingborough 1989.

    Louise Hay, *You Can Heal Your Life*, Eden Grove Editions, London 1988.

Appendix II

Useful Contacts (UK)

Physiotherapy
Therapists should be chartered and have the qualifications MCSP and SRP. For local practitioner contact:
> The Chartered Society of Physiotherapy,
> Tel: 020 7306 6666
> www.csp.org.uk

Osteopathy
Therapists should have the qualifications DO or BSc(Ost), and MRO. For local practitioner contact:
> General Council and Register of Osteopathy,
> Tel: 020 7357 66557
> www.osteopathy.org.uk

Chiropractic
Qualifications vary depending on where training took place. All those on the BCA register have undertaken a 5-year course of full-time study. For local practitioner contact:
> British Chiropractors Association,
> Tel: 0118 950 5950
> www.chiropractic-uk.co.uk

Alexander Technique
For list of registered teachers' names and addresses contact:
> The Society of Teachers in Alexander Technique (STAT),
> Tel: 0845 230 7828
> www.stat.org.uk

Feldenkrais Technique
For directory of teachers/practitioners and book list contact:
> Feldenkrais Guild UK,
> Tel: 07000 785506
> www.feldenkrais.co.uk

The RSI Association
Provides information and advice about Repetitive Strain Injuries.
> Tel helpline: 0800 018 5012
> www.rsi.org.uk

Disabled Living Foundation
Supplies domestic aids and equipment for people with disabilities.
> Tel helpline: 0845 130 9177
> www.dlf.org.uk

Back Shops
Suppliers of cushions and chairs designed for good posture, mail order service available.
> Tel: 020 7935 9120
> www.thebackshop.co.uk

Musicians' Benevolent Fund
May provide financial assistance to musicians with injuries.
> Tel: 020 7636 4481
> www.mbf.org.uk

BPAMT – British Performing Arts Medicine Trust
Provides advice and access to specialist medical consultation.
> Tel helplines: 020 7240 4500 (London)
>   0845 602 0235 (elsewhere in UK)
> www.bpamt.co.uk

ISSTIP – International Society for the Study of Tension in Performance
A Performing Arts Clinic is regularly held in London, and conferences and workshops are organised from time to time.
> Tel: 020 7373 7307
> www.musiciansgallery.com